theclinics.com

# CLINICS IN LIVER DISEASE

## Hepatocellular Carcinoma

GUEST EDITOR
Morris Sherman, MS BCh, PhD, FRCP(C)

CONSULTING EDITOR
Norman Gitlin, MD

May 2005 • Volume 9 • Number 2

SAUNDERS

An Imprint of Elsevier, Inc.
PHILADELPHIA LONDON TORONTO MONTREAL SYDNEY TOKYO

**W.B. SAUNDERS COMPANY**
*A Division of Elsevier Inc.*

The Curtis Center • Independence Square West • Philadelphia, Pennsylvania 19106

http://www.theclinics.com

**CLINICS IN LIVER DISEASE**
**May 2005**
Editor: Kerry Holland

**Volume 9, Number 2**
**ISSN 1089-3261**
**ISBN 1-4160-2779-3**



*Clinics in Liver Disease* (ISSN 1089-3261) is published quarterly by W.B. Saunders Company. Corporate and editorial offices: The Curtis Center, Independence Square West, Philadelphia, PA 19106-3399. Accounting and circulation offices: 6277 Sea Harbor Drive, Orlando, FL 32887-4800. Periodicals pending postage paid at Orlando, FL 32862, and additional mailing offices. Subscription prices are $165.00 per year (U.S. individuals), $83.00 per year (U.S. student/resident), $234.00 per year (U.S. institutions), $205.00 per year (foreign individuals), $103.00 per year (foreign student/resident), $273.00 per year (foreign institutions), $188.00 per year (Canadian individuals), and $273.00 per year (Canadian institutions). Foreign air speed delivery is included in all *Clinics* subscription prices. All prices are subject to change without notice. POSTMASTER: Send address changes to *Clinics in Liver Disease*, W.B. Saunders Company, Periodicals Fulfillment, Orlando, FL 32887-4800. **Customer Service: 1-800-654-2452** (US). From outside of the US, call **407-345-4000.** E-mail: hhspcs@harcourt.com.

Reprints. For copies of 100 or more, of articles in this publication, please contact the Commercial Reprints Department, Elsevier Inc., 360 Park Avenue South, New York, New York 10010-1710. Tel. (212) 633-3813 Fax: (212) 462-1935 e-mail: reprints@elsevier.com.

*Clinics in Liver Disease* is covered in *Index Medicus*.

Printed in the United States of America.

# CONSULTING EDITOR

**NORMAN GITLIN, MD,** Professor of Medicine, Atlanta Gastroenterology Associates, Crawford Long Hospital: An Emory Affiliate, Atlanta, Georgia

# GUEST EDITOR

**MORRIS SHERMAN, MS BCh, PhD, FRCP(C),** Assistant Professor of Medicine, University of Toronto; Toronto General Hospital, Toronto, Ontario, Canada

# CONTRIBUTORS

**ALEX S. BEFELER, MD,** Assistant Professor, Department of Internal Medicine, Division of Gastroenterology and Hepatology, Saint Louis University, St. Louis, Missouri

**F. XAVIER BOSCH, MD, PhD,** Unit Chief, Epidemiology and Cancer Registration Unit, IDIBELL, Institut Català d'Oncologia, L'Hospitalet de Llobregat, Barcelona, Spain

**CALOGERO CAMMÀ, MD,** Professor, Cattedra di Gastroenterologia, University of Palermo, Palermo, Italy; and IBIM, Consiglio Nazionale delle Ricerche, Palermo, Italy

**RAMON CLÉRIES, MSc,** Biostatistician, Epidemiology and Cancer Registration Unit, IDIBELL, Institut Català d'Oncologia, L'Hospitalet de Llobregat, Barcelona, Spain

**ANTONIO CRAXÌ, MD,** Professor, Cattedra di Gastroenterologia, University of Palermo, Palermo, Italy

**LAURA CROCETTI, MD,** Research Fellow, Department of Oncology, Transplants, and Advanced Technologies in Medicine, University of Pisa, Italy

**BRUNO DANIELE, MD, PhD,** Director, Medical Oncology Unit, "G. Rummo" Hospital Benevento, Italy

**MIREIA DÍAZ, BSc,** Biostatistician, Epidemiology and Cancer Registration Unit, IDIBELL, Institut Català d'Oncologia, L'Hospitalet de Llobregat, Barcelona, Spain

**HYUN-JUNG JANG, MD,** Assistant Professor, Department of Medical Imaging, Toronto General Hospital, University of Toronto, Toronto, Ontario, Canada

**TAE KYOUNG KIM, MD,** Associate Professor, Department of Medical Imaging, Toronto General Hospital, University of Toronto, Toronto, Ontario, Canada

**W. RAY KIM, MD, MBA,** Associate Professor of Medicine, Mayo Clinic College of Medicine, Division of Gastroenterology, Rochester, Minnesota

**RICCARDO LENCIONI, MD,** Associate Professor of Radiology, Department of Oncology, Transplants, and Advanced Technologies in Medicine, University of Pisa, Italy

**JOSEP M. LLOVET, MD,** Senior Visiting Scientist, Division of Liver Diseases, Recanati/Miller Transplantation Institute, Mount Sinai School of Medicine, New York, NY, USA; and BCLC Group, Liver Unit, Digestive Disease Institute, IDIABAPS, Hospital Clinic, University of Barcelona, Catalonia, Spain

**JORGE A. MARRERO, MD, MS,** Assistant Professor of Medicine, Division of Gastroenterology, University of Michigan, Ann Arbor, Michican, USA

**FRANCESCO PERRONE, MD, PhD,** Director, Clinical Trials Unit, National Cancer Institute, Napoli, Italy

**JOSEPA RIBES, MD,** Clinician, Epidemiology and Cancer Registration Unit, IDIBELL, Institut Català d'Oncologia, L'Hospitalet de Llobregat, Barcelona, Spain

**SASAN ROAYAIE, MD,** Assistant Professor, Recanati/Miller Transplantation Institute, Mount Sinai School of Medicine, New York, NY, USA

**IAN R. WANLESS, MD, FRCPC,** Department of Pathology, The Toronto Hospital, Toronto Canada

**STEPHANIE R. WILSON, MD,** Professor, Department of Medical Imaging, Toronto General Hospital, University of Toronto, Toronto, Ontario, Canada

# CONTENTS



Year 2000 estimates of the incidence of cancer indicate that primary liver cancer remains the fifth most common malignancy in men and the eighth in women. The number of new cases has been predicted as 564,000, corresponding to 398,000 in men and 166,000 in women. The geographic areas at highest risk are located in Eastern Asia, Middle Africa, and some countries of Western Africa. Changes in incidence among migrant populations underline the predominant role of environmental factors in the etiology of primary liver cancer. In high-risk countries, the early cases of primary liver cancer occur already at ages 20 and above, underlying the impact of viral exposures early in life. In countries at low risk, primary liver cancer is rare before the 50s, translating the impact of late exposures with moderate risks and long latency intervals. Sex ratios are typically between 2 and 4. The incidence of primary liver cancer is increasing in several developed countries including the United States, and the increase will likely continue for several decades. The trend has a dominant cohort effect related to exposures to hepatitis B and C viruses. The variability of primary liver cancer incidence is largely explained by the distribution and the natural history of the hepatitis B and C viruses. The attributable risk estimates for the combined effects of these infections account for well over 80% of liver cancer cases worldwide. Primary liver cancer is the first human cancer largely amenable to prevention using hepatitis B virus vaccines and screening of blood and blood products for hepatitis B and C viruses.

## FORTHCOMING ISSUES

August 2005

**Hepatitis C Virus**
Emmet B. Keeffe, MD, *Guest Editor*

November 2005

**Recent Advances in the Treatment of Liver Disorders**
Jorge Herrera, MD, *Guest Editor*

February 2006

**Pediatric Hepatology**
William Balisteri, MD, and
Jorge Bezerra, MD, *Guest Editors*

## RECENT ISSUES

February 2005

**Alcoholic Liver Disease**
Caroll B. Leevy, MD, *Guest Editor*

November 2004

**Metabolic Liver Diseases**
Bruce R. Bacon, MD, *Guest Editor*

August 2004

**Nonalcoholic Fatty Liver Disease**
Arun J. Sanyal, MBBS, MD, *Guest Editor*

May 2004

**Hepatitis B**
Tram T. Tran, MD, and
Paul Martin, MD, *Guest Editors*

ELSEVIER
SAUNDERS

CLINICS IN
LIVER DISEASE

Clin Liver Dis 9 (2005) xi–xii

Preface

# Hepatocellular Carcinoma

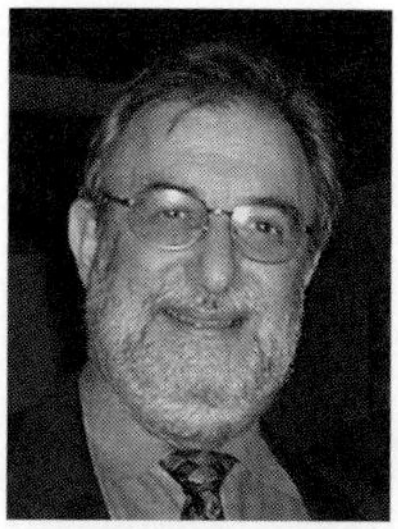

Morris Sherman, MS BCh, PhD, FRCP(C)
*Guest Editor*

In North America and Europe over the last 10 years or so, hepatocellular carcinoma (HCC) has become a much more common disease than in the past and is demanding more attention from clinicians. Along with this increase in incidence has come the realization that very little was known about HCC. A decade ago there were very few randomized controlled trials of therapy, the efficacy of screening was unknown (though it was presumed to be present), and little was known about the pathogenesis of this disease. Staging systems were rudimentary and had been developed without the appropriate statistical tools. Since then, the medical literature dealing with HCC has expanded considerably, and many studies have been conducted with increasing rigor; consequently, there is now some solid information in at least some aspects of this disease.

HCC has become very topical. The first international consensus conference on HCC management was in 2001, sponsored by the European Association for the Study of the Liver. A follow-up conference is due in 2005. In 2003 the American Association for the Study of Liver Diseases hosted a single-topic research symposium on HCC, and in 2004 the National Institutes of Health also held a research symposium on HCC. This issue of the *Clinics in Liver Disease* thus continues a trend of highlighting the importance of this disease for patients who have underlying liver disease.

This issue attempts to present some of the new information about HCC that has emerged over the last few years. Dr. Bosch and his colleagues describe the

1089-3261/05/$ – see front matter 
doi:10.1016/j.cld.2005.03.001

epidemiology of this disease and highlight how the incidence is increasing in parts of the world where it was previously considered to be a low-incidence disease. Drs. Daniele and Perrone discuss the difference between staging and scoring systems for HCC and describe current prognostic systems. Dr. Kim presents alternative ways of looking at disease in the absence of solid evidence by using modeling techniques. Screening for HCC remains controversial. Dr. Marrero clarifies some of the issues around the use of screening tests, particularly serologic screening tests, and indicates where in the development process these tests are. Imaging of HCC is crucial to both screening and to management. Dr. Wilson and colleagues present a discussion of the radiological features of HCC and present new information about the use of contrast-enhanced ultrasonography, a tool surely destined to be very useful in the management of this disease. The other diagnostic modality is of course biopsy, and Dr. Wanless discusses the difficulties in differentiating malignant from nonmalignant tissue in small lesions found on screening. There is a difference in interpretation between Japanese pathologists and Western pathologists as to where the dividing line between malignant and nonmalignant lies, and this is also discussed.

There are three articles devoted to therapy for HCC, including an assessment of embolization and chemoembolization by Dr. Befeler, of local ablative therapies by Dr. Lencioni and of transplantation for HCC beyond the usual criteria by Drs. Roayaie and Llovet. Finally, Dr. Craxi and Camma discuss prevention of HCC.

All the authors have been selected for their expertise in the areas described in their respective articles. It is the hope of the editors that the information presented here will be helpful to readers in understanding important aspects of the management of HCC. Just as important, we hope that this information highlights what we do not know as much as what we do know, and that it points the way to further studies.

Morris Sherman, MS BCh, PhD, FRCP(C)
*Toronto General Hospital, 9N–981*
*200 Elizabeth Street*
*Toronto, Ontario M5G 2C4, Canada*
*E-mail address:* morris.sherman@uhn.on.ca

ELSEVIER
SAUNDERS

Clin Liver Dis 9 (2005) 191–211

CLINICS IN
LIVER DISEASE

# Epidemiology of Hepatocellular Carcinoma

F. Xavier Bosch, MD, PhD*, Josepa Ribes, MD, Ramon Cléries, MSc, Mireia Díaz, BSc

*Epidemiology and Cancer Registration Unit, IDIBELL, Institut Català d'Oncologia, Avda. Gran Via s/n, Km 2.7, 08907 L'Hospitalet de Llobregat, Barcelona, Spain*

The epidemiology of hepatocellular carcinoma can be best evaluated through the use of national cancer registries, which generally list this tumor among those designated as "primary liver cancer." Therefore, the term "primary liver cancer" (PLC) will be used throughout this article.

## Incidence of liver cancer

For the year 2000 it has been estimated that some 564,000 new cases of PLC occurred worldwide, corresponding to 398,364 in men and 165,972 in women.

Table 1 presents the estimated number of cases per year and age-adjusted incidence and mortality rates of PLC worldwide by sex and geographic area. The table presents a combined analysis of the reports of the population-based cancer registries [1] and the World Health Organization mortality databank [2]. PLC accounts for 5.6% of all human cancers (7.5% among men and 3.5% among women) [1].

Fig. 1 shows the number of PLC cases in both sexes and plots the distribution of the age-adjusted incidence rates (AAIRs) as annual averages per 100,000 men [1,3]. The corresponding distribution of AAIRs among women follows a similar geographic pattern. The standard population used for the adjustment is the world standard, which tends to increase rates in countries with young populations and to decrease rates in countries with older populations.

Partial support has been received from the Instituto de Salud Carlos III of the Spanish Government (Grants RTICCC C03/09 and RTICESP C03/10).

* Corresponding author.

*E-mail address:* x.bosch@ico.scs.es (F.X. Bosch).

1089-3261/05/$ – see front matter 
doi:10.1016/j.cld.2004.12.009

***liver.theclinics.com***

Table 1
Estimated number of new cases and deaths, and incidence and mortality rates of primary liver cancer by geographical area

| | Incidence | | | | Mortality | | | |
|---|---|---|---|---|---|---|---|---|
| | Men | | Women | | Men | | Women | |
| Geographical area | N | AAIRs | N | AAIRs | N | AAMRs | N | AAMRs |
| World | 398.364 | 14,97 | 165.972 | 5,51 | 383.593 | 14,41 | 164.961 | 5,46 |
| Developed countries | 73.270 | 8,71 | 33.680 | 2,86 | 68.992 | 8,07 | 36.657 | 3,01 |
| Developing countries | 325.108 | 17,43 | 132.298 | 6,77 | 314.611 | 16,86 | 128.305 | 6,57 |
| Africa | | | | | | | | |
| Eastern | 8.476 | 14,44 | 4.003 | 6,02 | 8.313 | 14,17 | 3.929 | 5,91 |
| Middle | 6.672 | 24,21 | 4.280 | 12,98 | 6.539 | 23,73 | 4.195 | 12,72 |
| Northern | 2.583 | 4,95 | 1.577 | 2,68 | 2.529 | 4,85 | 1.547 | 2,63 |
| Southern | 839 | 6,16 | 357 | 2,07 | 784 | 5,80 | 336 | 1,95 |
| Western | 8.796 | 13,51 | 4.205 | 6,16 | 8.220 | 12,72 | 3.927 | 5,79 |
| Asia | | | | | | | | |
| Eastern | 271.527 | 35,46 | 101.909 | 12,66 | 257.046 | 33,50 | 97.485 | 12,09 |
| South-Eastern | 33.460 | 18,35 | 11.660 | 5,70 | 31.512 | 17,35 | 10.942 | 5,37 |
| South-Central | 14.677 | 2,77 | 8.055 | 1,45 | 14.400 | 2,72 | 7.884 | 1,41 |
| Western | 3.541 | 5,60 | 1.417 | 2,06 | 3.489 | 5,51 | 1.378 | 2,01 |
| Europe | | | | | | | | |
| Eastern | 10.568 | 5,80 | 7.360 | 2,55 | 10.842 | 5,91 | 8.142 | 2,76 |
| Northern | 1.915 | 2,61 | 1.326 | 1,39 | 2.167 | 2,86 | 1.660 | 1,64 |
| Southern | 11.647 | 9,84 | 5.571 | 3,45 | 12.235 | 10,09 | 7.150 | 4,27 |
| Western | 8.418 | 5,85 | 3.090 | 1,61 | 9.874 | 6,69 | 4.344 | 2,09 |
| America | | | | | | | | |
| Caribbean | 1.282 | 7,58 | 797 | 4,17 | 1.312 | 7,80 | 864 | 4,51 |
| Central | 878 | 2,06 | 786 | 1,64 | 910 | 2,14 | 820 | 1,70 |
| Southern | 6.110 | 4,80 | 5.597 | 3,68 | 6.031 | 4,75 | 5.592 | 3,67 |
| Northern[a] | 8.202 | 4,11 | 4.333 | 1,68 | 8.554 | 4,20 | 5.097 | 1,89 |
| Oceania | | | | | | | | |
| Australia and New Zealand | 541 | 3,60 | 212 | 1,19 | 529 | 3,45 | 252 | 1,37 |
| Pacific Islands[b] | 436 | 18,30 | 241 | 9,40 | 407 | 17,20 | 224 | 8,8 |

*Abbreviations:* AAIRs, Age-adjusted incidence rates; AAMRs, age-adjusted mortality rates.

[a] United States and Canada.

[b] Melanesia, Micronesia, and Polinesia.

Source: Globocan 2000, World Health Organization. Mortality Database 2001.

Fig. 2 shows the estimated AAIRs values among men for the 18 standard regions of the world and the corresponding box and whiskers [1,3]. In Eastern Asia, PLC AAIRs in males range from a relatively low AAIRs in Japan (29.21 per 100,000), to the high rates in Korea (48.77 per 100,000) and Mongolia (98.93 per 100,000). In Middle Africa, rates range from the low rates in Angola (5.77 per 100,000), to the high rates in Congo (32.33 per 100,000) with several registries reporting intermediate rates in Cameroon (17.72 per 100,000), Congo Brazzaville (13.24 per 100,000), and Gabon (13.01 per 100,000), and higher rates in Central African Republic (24.21 per 100,000) and Equatorial Guinea (24.21

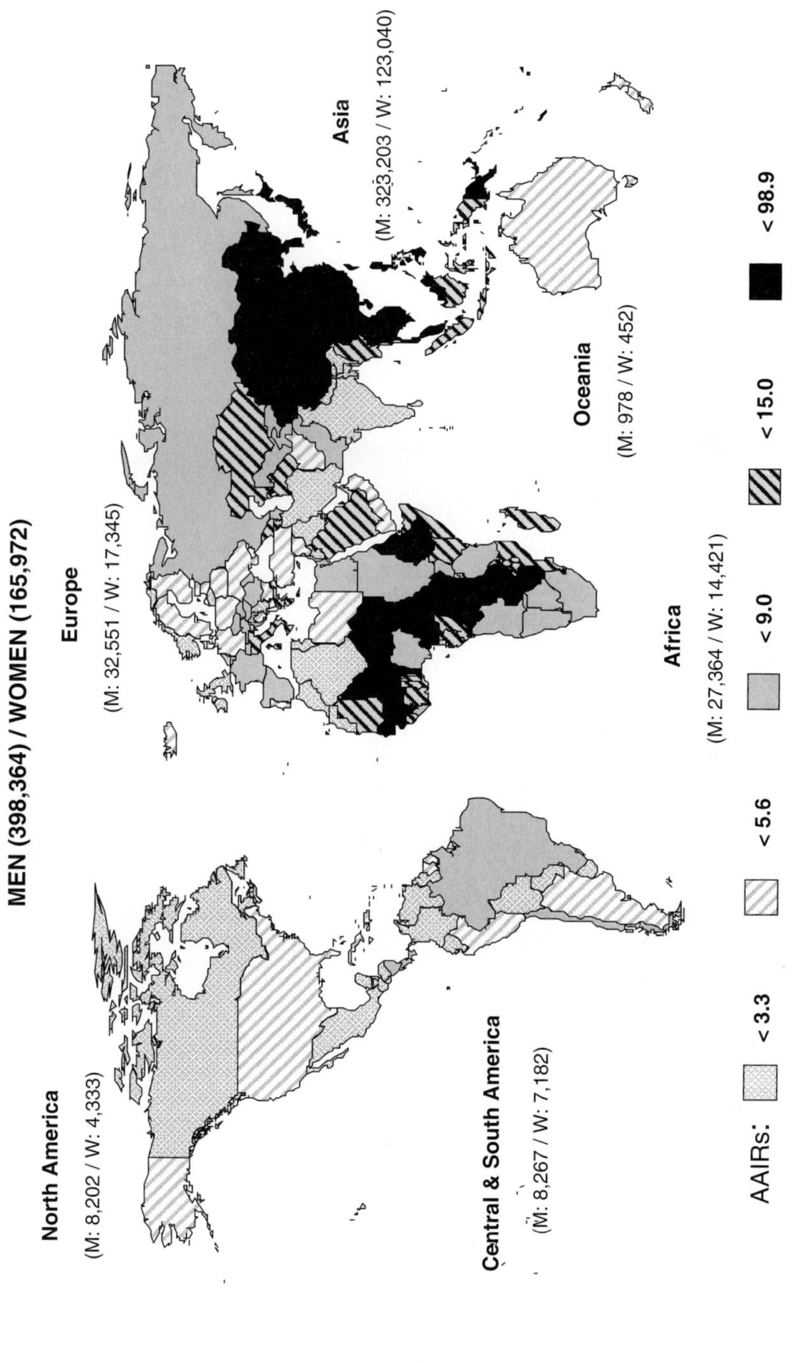


Fig. 1. Number of cases by world's region and age-adjusted incidence rates of PLC among men. Estimates for the year 2000.

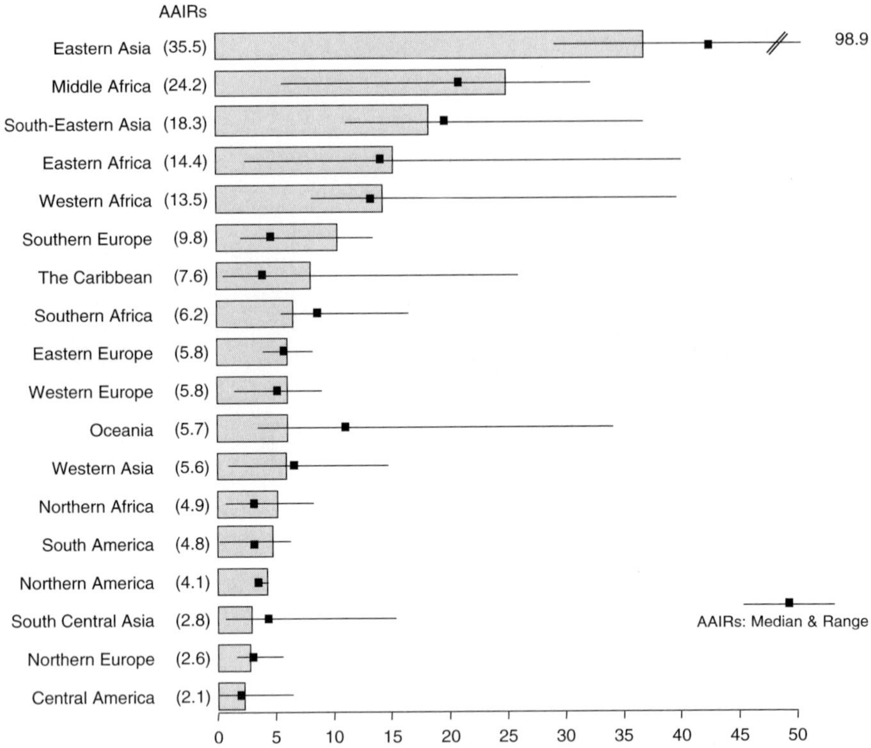


Fig. 2. Estimated age-adjusted incidence rates of PLC in men by geographical regions and their variability for the year 2000.

per 100,000). In Western Africa, incidence rates include low risk areas in Nigeria (8.20 per 100,000), and very high rates in The Gambia (39.67 per 100,000), Mali (34.56 per 100,000), and Guinea (33.15 per 100,000). This variability is also observed among women. In Australia and New Zealand, Europe, and the Americas the incidence is consistently below 10 per 100,000 and the intercountry variability in PLC incidence is lower.

## Age-specific incidence rates

In most high-risk areas, such as South-East Asia (Qidong in China) or the West Coast of Africa (Bamako in Mali), PLC rates increase after 20 years of age and peak or stabilize at the age intervals 50 and above (Fig. 3). In these countries PLC is not a rare event at ages 20 to 35. Still, the incidence in Qidong is substantially higher at each age group than the corresponding incidence in Mali, a high-risk country in Africa, and the mean age of occurrence is significantly shifted toward the young age groups [3,4].

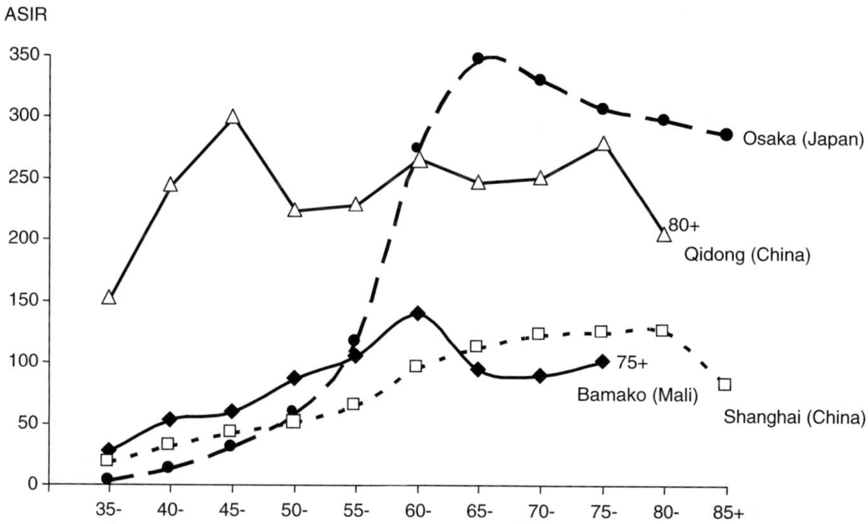


Fig. 3. Age-specific incidence rates of PLC in men in selected high-risk populations.

A second pattern is observed in high-risk countries with recent substantial degrees of development. For example, in the cancer registry in Shanghai, rates are lower than the corresponding rates in Qidong, and the age-specific incidence increases steadily with age, a pattern similar to the one usually observed in low-risk areas. In the Osaka Cancer Registry in Japan, the incidence among men increases after the age range 45 to 50, and reaches a plateau in the 65 and above years of age [4].

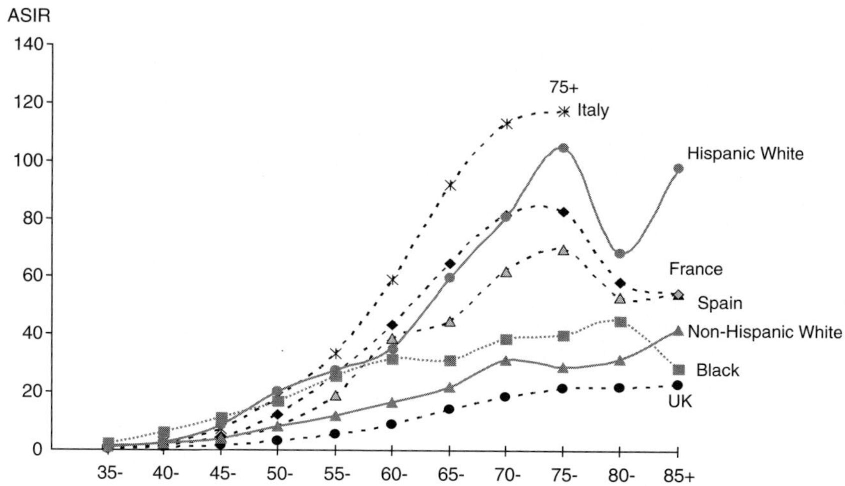


Fig. 4. Age-specific incidence rates of PLC in men in selected populations in Europe and in the United States.

Fig. 4 shows the age-specific incidence rates among men in selected European countries and ethnic groups in the United States. The global higher risk in the Mediterranean countries in Europe is reflected in all age groups, most notably in the elderly. The age-specific pattern among non-Hispanic White populations in the United States is similar to the one registered in Europe. Hispanic Whites in the United States show a peculiar trend with steep increases after age 60, without a clear explanation on the risk factors that operate in these groups of older migrants [3,4].

The age-specific incidence rates also reflect the differences in the natural history of hepatitis B virus (HBV) and hepatitis C virus (HCV)-related PLC cases. In Korea, for example, the mean age at onset of the HBV-related PLC is around 55, which is 10 years younger than the average age at onset of HCV-related PLC cases [5].

## Sex ratios

The correlation between AAIRs PLC in men and women is extremely high in 157 registries worldwide: correlation coefficient [CC] = 0.953, $P < 0.001$) [6]. An excess of PLC incidence among men compared with women has been well

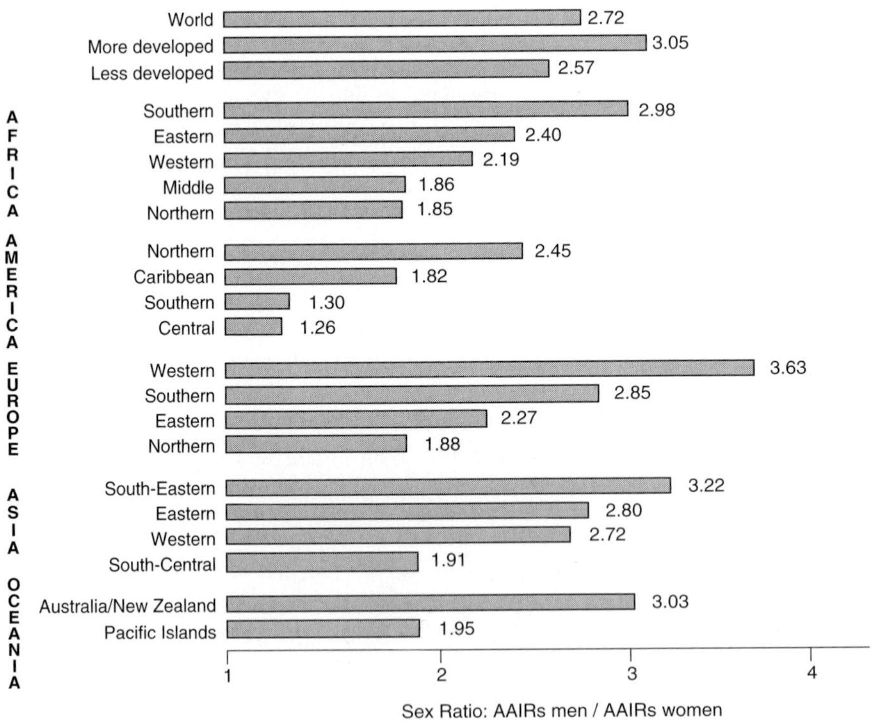


Fig. 5. Sex ratio in PLC incidence by geographical area.

documented. Worldwide, the range of the ratios in the sex-specific AAIRs is 1.3 to 3.6 (Fig. 5) [1]. In high-risk countries, sex ratios tend to be higher, and the male excess is more pronounced below 50 years of age. Migrant populations also show a shift in the sex ratio values. Japanese populations in the United States show a fairly steady sex ratio between 2 and 3 in the age groups above 50, whereas Japanese populations in Japan show excess risk between 3 and 5 in the same age groups. In the age groups below 50, the sex ratios of PLC among Japanese in Japan range between 7 and 10. Among Japanese in the United States, the incidence of PLC among women below age 50 is too rare, and the sex ratio calculations are unreliable [4]. In populations with low incidence, the highest sex ratios occur later, in the 60 to 70 years of age group [7].

The biologic interpretation of the sex ratio observations has not been satisfactory proven. Several hypothesis have been investigated, including the interaction of testosterone with the HBV cycle or the impact of sex specific exposures such as alcohol or tobacco in some cultural environments [8,9].

## Mortality from liver cancer

Coding recommendations of PLC and liver metastasis changed slightly from the eighth to the ninth revisions of the International Classification of Diseases (ICD) implemented after 1965 and 1975, respectively [10,11]. The 10th revision was introduced as from 1992 [12].

The description of the codes for PLC (155.0 in the eighth and ninth ICD versions) as well as for liver cirrhosis (571 in the eighth and ninth ICD versions) has not changed across these two classifications. The 10th Revision of the ICD introduced a major change (C22.0 for PLC and K74 for liver cirrhosis). The eighth Revision differentiated the diagnoses of "liver metastases" (197.7) and liver cancer (LC) "unknown if primary or metastatic" (197.8). The ninth revision incorporated a new code for cancers in the liver "unknown if primary or metastatic" (155.2) that largely superimposed the 197.8 category in the eighth ICD. The 10th revision kept the same concept of liver cancer "unknown if primary or metastatic" with a new code (C22.9). It also clarified the histology of the liver cancer tumors (hepatocellular carcinoma = C22.0, biliary tract intrahepatic = C22.1, liver cancer unknown origin = C22.9, hepatoblastoma = C22.2, angiosarcoma = C22.3, other sarcoma = C22.4, and other specific hepatic carcinomas = C22.7). Therefore, if properly done, in countries with developed health systems the predictable impact of changing codes for liver cancer should be, if any, of a small reduction in incidence as a result of decreasing the number of liver metastasis misclassified as PLC. For the majority of high-risk countries, the relative impact of the diagnostic ability, including access to medical care as well as technology, should be considerably more important than the variability attributed to coding practices.

Another source of variability of the health statistics is the intercountry differences with regard to the number of entries from death certificates that are routinely extracted and coded. In some countries, several diagnosis are processed and additional rules apply in the assignment of the cause of death [13]. This is particularly important in PLC because of the high frequency of concurrent liver cirrhosis (over 90% in most populations) and its clinical complications, many of which can lead to an immediate cause of death. These sources of variability should particularly be considered when time trends are calculated and international comparisons are to be made.

Despite the limitations of mortality data, PLC age-adjusted mortality rates (AAMRs) follow a geographic pattern consistent with the incidence data (Table 1) [1,2]. PLC is a tumor with high lethality and a yearly fatality ratio around 1, indicating that most cases do not survive a year. In Europe, for the period 1990 to 1999 [14], and in the United States for the period 1995 to 2000 [15], PLC survival rates at the population level were analyzed from the unselected data of population-based cancer registries. The 5-year relative survival rate (mortality from PLC adjusted for mortality from competing causes) was 6.5% and 8.3%, respectively. There are few differences in survival rates according to sex, suggesting a similar distribution of stage at diagnosis. In developing countries PLC is inevitably fatal.

## Primary liver cancer in ethnic groups and migrant populations

Cancer registries in the United States report on the incidence of PLC by ethnic origin in populations with similar exposures to environmental risk factors. The lowest incidence rates are consistently found among Caucasian Whites (3.8 in men and 1.4 in women). Gradually increasing rates are found in Japanese (5.5 in men and 4.3 in women), Black (7.1 in men and 2.1 in women), Hispanic White (9.8 in men and 3.5 in women), Filipino (10.9 in men and 2.4 in women), Chinese (16.2 in men and 5.0 in women), and Korean (20.7 in men and 10.4 in women). Among women, the high-risk ethnic groups present two- to fivefold higher PLC AAIRs than the rates observed in non-Hispanic White women [4]. These cross-sectional rates are consistent with some genetically determined susceptibility to PLC across ethnic groups. Migrant studies have been instrumental in the evaluation of the relative contribution of environmental and genetically determined host factors in PLC [16]. Several studies have been conducted among migrant populations comparing their PLC mortality rates to the rates of the host population. Table 2 summarizes most of the published studies in which country of origin is usually a high risk area and the host population is taken as reference [17–22]. Among men, a 1.3- to 10.9-fold excess of PLC mortality is observed among Asian migrants to North America, Australia, or Europe. A 31.6-fold higher risk has been reported among West African migrants to England and Wales and a 5.3-fold higher mortality rates among Caribbean migrants. Among women, perhaps due to the small number of death cases, the results of these studies are not as consistent, and the excess of PLC mortality among migrants ranges from 1.1- to fivefold [17–22].

Some of these studies have demonstrated that the risk of dying from PLC weakens in the migrant's descendants and in migrants living for a long time in the

Table 2
Relative risks of primary liver cancer in migrant populations compared to host populations

| Host region | Region of origin | Range RR men | Range RR women | RR both sexes |
|---|---|---|---|---|
| US | China | 3.3–10.9 | 1.1–4.3 | — |
| Canada | China | 7.7–10.5 | 2.5–3.0 | — |
| Australia | China | 5.2 | 2.6 | — |
| | East Asia | — | — | 8.9 |
| | Southeast Asia | — | — | 10.0 |
| | Near East | 2.5 | 0.3 | — |
| France | East Asia | 1.3 | 3.3 | — |
| | Southeast Asia | 2.5 | 1.6 | — |
| England and Wales | West African | 31.6 | 5.4 | — |
| | East African | 1.1 | 1.8 | — |
| | Caribbean | 5.3 | 3.2 | — |

*Abbreviation:* RR, relative risk.
*Adapted from* Bosch et al., [3].
Source: [17–22].

host country. In the United States, King and Locke [23] estimated the risk of dying from PLC in two generations of Asian migrants, finding a remarkable attenuation in the magnitude of the estimates. Excess mortality rates were 10.9 in the first and 2.8 in the second generation among men and 5.2 and 2.1 among women. A study conducted in Australia found a substantial reduction of the risk of dying from PLC among East and South-East Asian migrants according to duration of residence: 12.1 for 0 to 9 years of residence, 11.9 for 10 to 19 years, 5.0 for 20 to 29 years, and 3.1 for more than 30 years [22]. In the United States, a study based on PLC incidence confirmed these results. PLC AAIRs in Chinese, Japanese, and Filipino migrants to the United States and their descendants were compared with PLC AAIRs of US-born Whites. In this study, rates of PLC were consistently higher for Asian men born in Asia than those of Asian men born in the United States (second generations or more) as follows: Chinese born in China: 26.5; Chinese born in the United States: 9.8; Japanese born in Japan: 16.5; Japanese born in the United States: 6.6; Filipinos born in The Philippines: 11.4 and Filipinos born in the United States: 6.5. The comparison incidence rate for the United States Whites was 3.4. Among Asian American women, the trends were not as consistent (Asian-born and US-born women showed incidence rates as follows: Chinese: 2.2 and 3.7; Japanese: 1.9 and 1.4; Filipino: 2.6 and 0.0, and the referent point corresponded to the United States Whites: 1.1) [24].

## Trends in liver cancer incidence and mortality

International variation in the diagnostic ability as well as in the coding and registration practices for PLC (primary, intrahepatic biliary ducts, metastases, and liver tumors of uncertain nature as if primary or secondary) makes the interpretation of long-term time trends difficult. Of particular concern in some countries is the likely impact of migrants from high-risk countries. These populations are often visible in the health system at the time of diagnosis, and are less likely to be counted in the census and still constitute an important component of the number of PLC cases [17–22].

During the last 2 decades, increases of PLC incidence rates have been reported in Australia, Central Europe [25,26], the United Kingdom [27], Japan [28], and North America [29,30]. Decreasing trends were reported from Chinese populations in Singapore and Shanghai, India, Sweden, and Spain [26].

Several reports from the United States population have investigated the consistency in trends using three different sources of information, namely liver cancer hospitalization rates, incidence rates from Cancer Registries, and mortality rates from the United States population. The studies covered a time period from 1976 to 2003 and, for the analyses of cancer incidence, it was possible to restrict the comparisons to the cases that showed histopathology confirmation of hepatocellular carcinoma (HCC) (about 75% of the reported cases). The study reported significant increasing trends for the Black, White, and Hispanic populations. The analyses of the components of the trends, suggested that, in the United States, there is a predominant cohort effect [29,30].

International trends in PLC mortality have also been evaluated. Among males, increases in mortality to PLC have been reported in the United States, Japan, Australia, Scotland, France, and Italy, while decreasing trends have been reported in the United Kingdom [31,32]. Trends among women are largely consistent. Increases in Cholangiocarcinoma have also been reported in the United States, Japan, England, and Wales, Australia, Spain, and Scotland, and among women in the United States, Australia, and England and Wales [31,33,34].

## Risk factors for primary liver cancer

The etiology of PLC has been largely established, and Table 3 shows current estimates of the attributable fractions for the main risk factors by three geographic areas [3].

Table 3
Risk factors of primary liver cancer and estimates of the attributable fractions (%)

| | Europe and US | | Japan | | Africa and Asia | |
|---|---|---|---|---|---|---|
| | Estimate | Range | Estimate | Range | Estimate | Range |
| Hepatitis B virus | 22 | 4–58 | 20 | 18–44 | 60 | 40–90 |
| Hepatitis C virus | 60 | 12–72 | 63 | 48–94 | 20 | 9–56 |
| Alcohol | 45 | 8–57 | 20 | 15–33 | — | 11–41 |
| Tobacco | 12 | 0–14 | 40 | 9–51 | 22 | — |
| Oral contraceptives | — | 10–50 | — | — | 8 | — |
| Aflatoxin | Limited exposure | | Limited exposure | | Important exposure | |
| Other risk factors | <5 | — | — | — | <5 | — |

Reproduced from Ref. [3].

## Hepatitis viruses

Overall, 75% to 80% of the PLC cases can be related to persistent viral infections with either HBV (50–55%) or HCV (25–30%). Worldwide, strong geographic correlations have been found between the incidence of PLC and the prevalences of hepatitis B suface anigen (HBsAg) (CC, 0.67, $P < 0.001$) or HCV antibody (anti-HCV) (CC, 0.37, $P < 0.001$) [6].

The role of chronic infection with HBV in the etiology of PLC is well established. Cohort studies conducted worldwide yielded relative risk estimates of 5.6 to 103.0, with the highest values reported from China and Taiwan (Table 4) [35–51]. Age at HBV infection is a key determinant of the risk. In developed areas at low risk of PLC, HBV acquisition at birth or during childhood is rare, and most of the viral infections are acquired in adolescence or adulthood, through sexual contacts, blood transfusions, or other invasive procedures under nonsterile conditions [52]. In these populations, the impact of cofactors such as alcohol and tobacco is reflected only in the incidence of PLC in the most advanced age groups. In contrast, mother-to-child transmission of HBV and HBV exposures in the first years of life are typical of most of the high-risk countries.

More specifically, one possible explanation for the differences in incidence rates in China and West Africa can be related to age at infection. In many Asian countries, there is a high prevalence of HBsAg carrier mothers who also express Hepatitis B "e" antigen (HBeAg) and remain HBV-DNA–positive throughout the reproductive age intervals [53–55]. In high-risk areas in Africa, the mother-to-child transmission rate is somehow lower and the child-to-child mode of transmission predominates. The impact of cofactors, perhaps with the exception of Aflatoxin, in the high-risk countries is likely to be marginal.

The reduction of risk observed in migrants to lower risk host populations probably reflects a combination of the reduction in the mother-to-child trans-

Table 4
Cohort studies among Hepatitis B virus carriers published since 1981: Primary liver cancer risk of death estimates

| | Range RR | Adjustment for other risk factors |
|---|---|---|
| U.S. | | |
| USA [35,36] | 9.7–26.8 | No |
| EUROPE | | |
| UK and Wales [37,38] | 26.3 | No |
| ASIA | | |
| Japan [39–44] | 5.6–21.0 | 1 study (alcohol and tobacco) |
| Taiwan [45–47] | 9.6–10.3 | 1 study (alcohol, tobacco, and HCV) |
| China [48–51] | 6.7–38.6 | 2 studies (alcohol, tobacco, and aflatoxins)<br>1 study (aflatoxins)<br>1 study (alcohol, tobacco, tea, LC family history, and occupational) |

*Abbreviations:* RR, relative risk; LC, liver cancer.

mission of HBV linked to mixing populations, the reduction of exposure to contaminated blood products during medical interventions or other invasive medical or ritual procedures, the lower prevalence of HBV (and possibly HCV) among siblings and, more recently, the impact of the massive introduction of HBV vaccines.

Iatrogenic exposures to HCV during massive public health interventions have been demonstrated, and the subsequent risk of PLC is now being expressed. Fig. 6 shows the prevalence of anti-HCV in three populations by age groups. The Japanese population, the United States population, and in the general population in Egypt [56,57]. The three graphs are consistent with predominant cohort effects. In Japan, increasing PLC incidence and mortality trends since the early 1970s have been related to exposure of the population to HCV through blood transfusion or contaminated needles in vaccination campaigns against tuberculoses and to intravenous drug use after World War II [57,58]. In Japan, the cross-sectional anti-HCV prevalence decreases with the youth of the cohort [57]. In the United States, the predominant cohort component of the increases in PLC incidence and mortality have been interpreted as a long-term consequence of important HCV exposure in the period 1960 to 1970 through contact with contaminated blood and syringe exchange in the relevant generations [59]. It is predictable that the number of PLC cases generated by the pool of HCV carriers will continue to increase for some time in the United States. The impact of the introduction of generalized HCV testing of blood products and the public awareness of the risks of HCV linked in part to the acquired immune deficiency

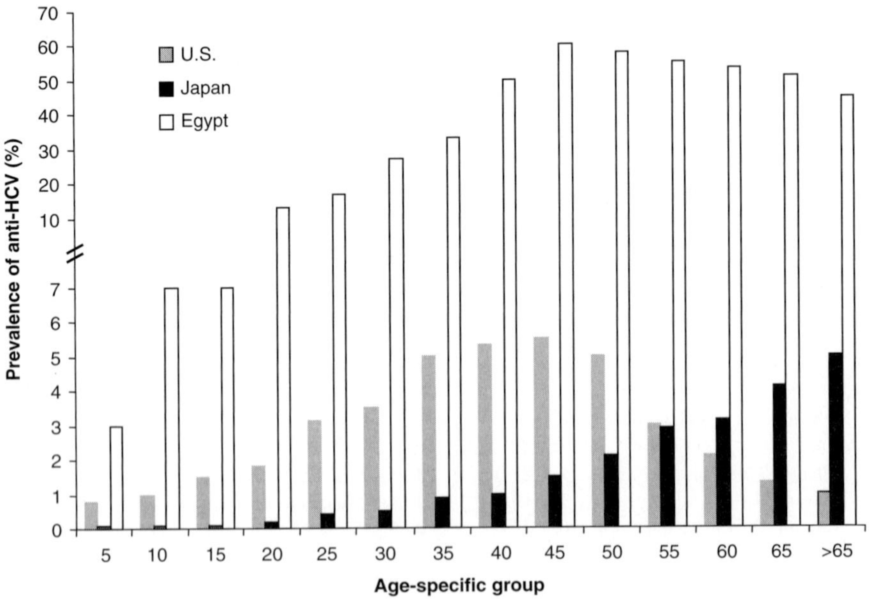


Fig. 6. HCV antibody seroprevalence by age groups in three countries.

syndrome (AIDS) education campaigns should result in lower HCV-related liver cancer in the more distant future.

In Egypt, a documented epidemiologic study traced the source of the infection to the massive treatment campaigns against schistosomal infestation conducted in the interval 1920 to 1970 of the general population. The treatment typically included several courses of intramuscular or intravenous drugs against schistosoma that were delivered under nonsterile conditions [60]. The anti-HCV prevalence in the population is one at the highest registered in all age groups (Fig. 6) [56].

Fig. 7 shows the impact of the two viral types in liver cancer in Japan and the United States. Fig. 7A shows the global increased number of deaths from PLC in the interval 1975 to 1992 in Japan. Although the prevalence of HBV-related PLC remains fairly constant over the period, the bulk of the increase seems to be related to HCV-linked PLC [61]. In the United States, the number of hospitalization PLC cases linked to HCV has increased dramatically compared with the HBV-related or alcohol-related PLC cases in the period 1993 to 1998 (Fig. 7B) [62].

More precise estimates of the relative contribution of viral infections to PLC incidence is being provided by the introduction of more advanced detection methods in epidemiologic studies. A review of the prevalence of HBsAg and of anti-HCV in PLC cases from various continents and the presence of HBV-DNA or HCV-RNA in cases of PLC that are negative for both serologic markers [63]. A large collaborative study in Europe, using Polymerase Chain Reaction (PCR) technology found that of the PLC cases that were negative for HBsAg or anti-HCV, an additional 33% were positive for HBV-DNA and 7% positive for HCV-RNA [64,65]. This observation has been repeatedly confirmed, and the trend suggests that in countries where HBV is common, the presence of HBV-DNA among HBsAg negative PLC cases is higher than the one found in European cases. A meta-analysis on viral factors and PLC reported summary odds ratios (OR) for HBsAg positivity without anti-HCV or HCV-RNA of 22.5 (95% confidence interval [CI], 19.5–26.0). The OR for anti-HCV/HCV-RNA positivity and HBsAg negativity was 17.3 (95% CI, 13.9–21.6), and the OR for positivity to HBV and HCV was OR: 165 (95% CI, 81.2–374), suggesting a synergism of the two viral infection in the causation of PLC [66,67].

The impact of the variants of HBV or HCV is now being described. There is substantial international variability on the prevalence of specific viral genotypes, and there is some evidence that genotypes may modulate the risk of progression to severe liver disease and probably PLC [68]. Of the HBV types described, type A is predominant in the United States and the Caribbean, type D in Europe and in the Middle East, and that types B and C predominate in Asia. In Africa, types A, C, and D are equally prevalent [69]. Within the United States, type A is more prevalent in the South, types C and B in the West, and type D is relatively more frequent in the Eastern parts of the country. Likewise, the prevalence of type 1b of HCV in PLC cases range from 50% in England and Germany to 70% to 90% in Italy and Spain [65].

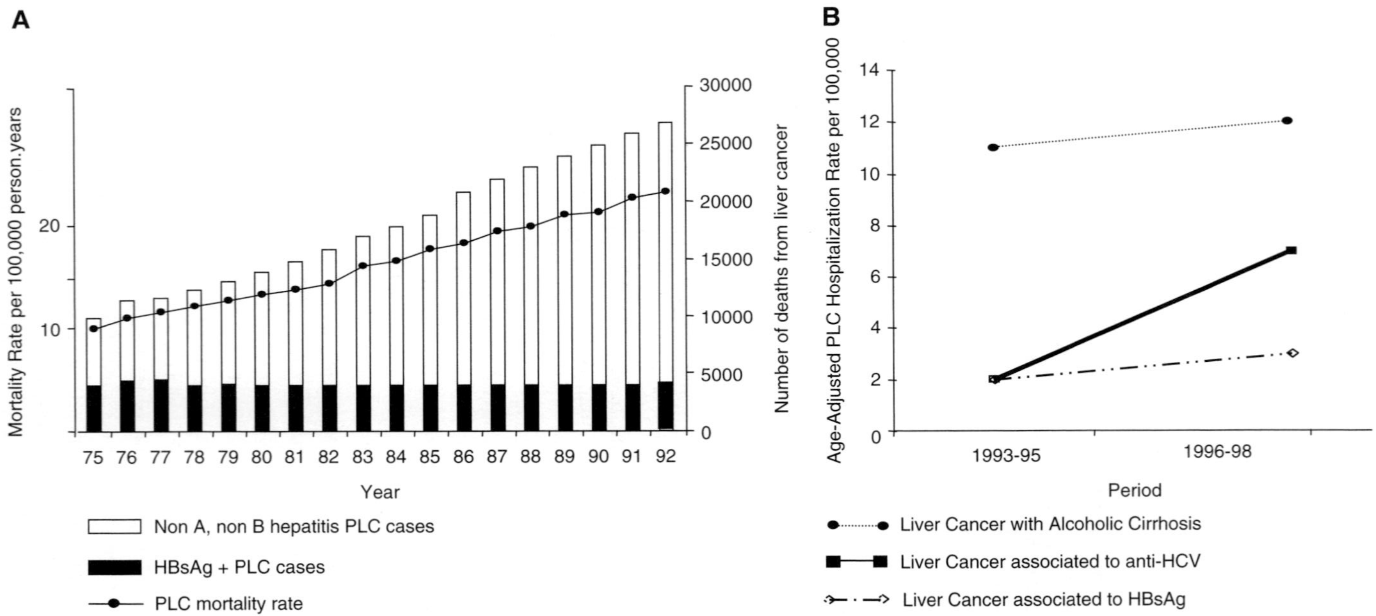


Fig. 7. (*A*) Time trends in liver cancer mortality rates in Japan by cause. (*B*) Temporal trends of the age-adjusted proportional hospitalization rates for PLC in the United States.

More research is warranted to describe how the natural history of the variants may affect viral spreading and carcinogenesis and, in more practical terms, its potential impact in modifying the response to the HBV vaccines currently employed.

## Aflatoxin

PLC has been related to aflatoxin exposures in human diets in countries where fungal infestation of crops and animal feed are common. Studies that used Aflatoxin/Albumin adducts, Aflatoxin M1 in urine, Aflatoxin-N7-Guanine adducts in urine, or p53-specific mutations (G to T transversions at codon 249), tend to indicate that individuals who are carriers of persistent HBV infection and who are exposed to aflatoxins in their diets have an increased risk of progression to PLC compared with non-Aflatoxin exposed HBV carriers. A similar interaction with chronic HCV has not been documented [70]. The evidence is, however, limited to a few studies and not consistent [53], and it has been difficult to document the impact of Aflatoxin exposure in the absence of viral infections.

## Alcohol and tobacco

Chronic alcohol abuse and alcoholic cirrhosis have long been recognized as a cause of PLC. However, it is not certain whether alcohol is a true carcinogen or if acts as a cofactor in the presence of coexistent infection with HBV or HCV. Several epidemiologic studies among alcoholics have described a high prevalence of HBV markers (16–70%) and of HCV markers (10–20%) compared with a background prevalence of close to 5% and less than 1%, respectively. These prevalences are even higher in PLC patients who are also alcoholics (27–81% of HBV markers and 50–77% of HCV markers), suggesting a complex interaction between alcohol and viral infections in the etiology of PLC [71]. Studies conducted in Northern Italy and Greece estimated that the attributable fraction (%) for high levels of alcohol consumption, once adjusted for HBV and HCV status were 45% in Italy [72] and 15% in Greece [73].

The association of cigarette smoking and PLC has been claimed from the results of some epidemiologic studies, notably in Japan. The evidence is, however, not consistent, and residual effects of nondetected HBV or HCV cannot be safely ruled out from the majority of the epidemiologic studies. Recent data from China and Taiwan have also reported an association of cigarette smoking with PLC independent of HBV status [74,75].

The sex-specific impact of alcohol, tobacco, and oral contraceptives (OC) use could explain the sex ratio pattern as well as the steady increase in incidence by age observed in the populations where these exposures are common.

## Hormonal factors

The occurrence of benign liver adenomas and occasional PLC among women who were long-term OC users has been documented. Several case–control studies conducted in developed countries where substantial number of women have used OC for extended periods of time have found risks between 1.6 and 5.5 among ever OC users, and a relationship with duration of use was observed in some of them [76]. In one of the few studies conducted in the Black population in South Africa, a country with high prevalence of HBV, no association between OC and PLC in women was found [77]. Analysis of the mortality trends for PLC in young women in the United Kingdom, the United States, Japan, and Sweden, provide no support for a measurable effect of OC on mortality due to PLC [78–80]. A multicentric study conducted with 317 cases of PLC among women under 65 years and 1060 controls found and association between this tumor and duration of OC use in the small subgroup of PLC cases without liver cirrhosis and with negative serology for HBV and HCV [81]. Further studies are needed to clarify and quantify the role of OC in PLC, an issue of considerable public health interest.

Other hormonal factors have been explored to explain the increased male susceptibility worldwide. A recent study in the United States found a protection linked to parity, late menopause, use of hormonal replacement therapy, and early age at menarchy. Except the latter, all factors were independent of HBV status [82]. Likewise, androgens have been postulated as a risk factor for PLC [9].

## Other risk factors and emerging factors

Other factors that may modulate the long-term impact of HBV or HCV persistent infections include dietary factors, some chemicals (such as arsenic), some hereditary conditions (hemochromatosis, Wilson's Disease, and other), and nutritional factors. Growing interest is currently focusing on the associations of PLC with diabetes mellitus [83–86], obesity, and the syndromes related to insulin resistance. Nonalcoholic fatty liver disease is being proposed as a risk factor for PLC [87]. Because of the considerable prevalence of some of these conditions in Western populations, it is of importance to conduct research to properly describe the nature of the associations observed.

## Prevention for primary liver cancer

By the year 2000, HBV vaccination programs had been implemented in 135 countries, including deprived areas in Africa and Asia. A major input from donor agencies has made it possible in the last decade, and such efforts should be encouraged and supported. HBV vaccination trials initiated in the 1980s have already shown the ability HBV vaccines to prevent the chronic carriage of

HBsAg [88,89] and the development of liver cancer when vaccination takes place at birth in Taiwan [90], or as adults among HBsAg negative men in Korea [91].

Screening of blood products for HCV markers in the countries that have introduced such programs has substantially reduced the rate of posttransfusion HCV infections [92]. Awareness of the negative impact of unprotected sex, important alcohol consumption, and smoking has probably had some impact in risk behavior modification. However, its potential impact on the incidence of PLC remains to be documented. Finally, the claim has been made that Aflatoxin reduction has reduced the incidence of PLC in Singapore and Shanghai, although final proof has not been provided.

## Summary

PLC remains a major health problem with great geographic variability. Men are consistently more affected than women, and survival is poor worldwide. Increasing trends in incidence in some developed countries including the United States suggest an underlying cohort effect linked to HCV and HBV exposures. Reduction of PLC burden in most developing countries should give priority to HBV vaccination campaigns and to prevention of HBV and HCV contamination. This implies reinforcing control of blood and derivatives, as well as the use of sterile medical equipment. HBV chronic carries may further benefit from reductions in the aflatoxin exposure in their diets. If achieved, aflatoxin reduction may also offer some protection to HCV carriers. In low-risk populations, alcohol consumption may account for the majority of the PLC cases that do not show viral markers.

## Acknowledgments

The authors wish to acknowledge with gratitude the support of Cristina Rajo in the preparation of the manuscript.

## References

[1] Ferlay J, Bray F, Pisani P, et al. Globocan 2000: cancer incidence, mortality and prevalence worldwide. Version 1.0. Lyon: IARC Press; 2001.

[2] World Health Organization. Mortality database. WHO statistical information system; 2001. Available at: http://www.who.int/whosis. Accessed June, 2001.

[3] Bosch FX, Ribes J, Díaz M, et al. Primary liver cancer: worldwide incidence and trends. Gastroenterology 2004;127(5 Suppl 1):S5–16.

[4] Parkin DM, Whelan SL, Ferlay J, et al, editors. Cancer incidence in five continents. Volume VIII. IARC Scientific Publications No. 155. Lyon: International Agency for Research on Cancer; International Association of Cancer Registries; 2002.

[5] Lee HS, Han CJ, Kim CY. Predominant etiologic association of hepatitis C virus with hepatocellular carcinoma compared with hepatitis B virus in elderly patients in a hepatitis B-endemic area. Cancer 1993;72(9):2564–7.
[6] Bosch FX, Ribes J, Borras J. Epidemiology of primary liver cancer. Semin Liver Dis 1999;19(3): 271–85.
[7] Bosch FX. Global epidemiology of hepatocellular carcinoma. In: Okuda K, Tabor E, editors. Liver cancer. London: Churchill Livingstone; 1997. p. 13–28.
[8] Donato F, Tagger A, Gelatti U, et al. Alcohol and Hepatocellular carcinoma: the effect of lifetime intake and hepatitis virus infections in men and women. Am J Epidemiol 2002;155(4): 323–31.
[9] Yu MW, Yang YC, Yang SY, et al. Hormonal markers and hepatitis B virus-related hepatocellular carcinoma risk: a nested case-control study among men. J Natl Cancer Inst 2001;93(21): 1644–51.
[10] World Health Organization. International classification of diseases. 8th Revision (ICD-8). Geneva: WHO; 1967.
[11] World Health Organization. International classification of diseases. 9th Revision (ICD-9). Geneva: WHO; 1977.
[12] World Health Organization. International classification of diseases. 10th Revision (ICD-10). Geneva: WHO; 1992.
[13] Hoel DG, Ron E, Carter R, et al. Influence of death certificate errors on cancer mortality trends. J Natl Cancer Inst 1993;85(13):1063–8.
[14] Coleman MP, Gatta G, Verdecchia A, et al. EUROCARE-3 summary: cancer survival in Europe at the end of the 20th century. Ann Oncol 2003;14(Suppl 5):V128–49.
[15] Ries LAG, Eisner MP, Kosary CL, et al. SEER Cancer Statistics Review, 1975–2001. Bethesda, MD: National Cancer Institute; 2004. Available at: http://seer.cancer.gov/csr/1975_2001/results_merged/topic_survival.pdf. Accessed July, 2004.
[16] Parkin DM. Studies of cancer in migrant populations: methods and interpretation. Rev Epidemiol Sante Publique 1992;40(6):410–24.
[17] Hanley AJ, Choi BC, Holowaty EJ. Cancer mortality among Chinese migrants: a review. Int J Epidemiol 1995;24:255–65.
[18] Khlat M, Bouchardy C, Parkin DM. Cancer mortality in immigrants from the Near East in Australia. Rev Epidemiol Sante Publique 1993;41(3):208–17.
[19] Bouchardy C, Parkin DM, Khlat M. Cancer moratlity among Chinese and South-East Asian migrants in France. Int J Cancer 1994;58:638–43.
[20] Fang J, Madhavan S, Alderman MH. Cancer mortality of Chinese in New York City 1988–1992. Int J Epidemiol 1996;25:907–12.
[21] Grulich AE, Swerdlow AJ, Head J, et al. Cancer mortality in African and Caribbean migrants to England and Wales. Br J Cancer 1992;66:905–11.
[22] McCredie M, Williams S, Coates M. Cancer mortality in East and Southeast Asian migrants to New South Wales, Australia, 1975–1995. Br J Cancer 1999;79:1277–82.
[23] King H, Locke FB. Cancer mortality among Chinese in the United States. J Natl Cancer Inst 1980;65(5):1141–8.
[24] Rosenblatt KA, Weiss NS, Schwartz SM. Liver cancer in Asian migrants to the United States and their descendants. Cancer Causes Control 1996;7(3):345–50.
[25] Benhamiche AM, Faivre C, Minello A, et al. Time trends and age-period-cohort effects on the incidence of primary liver cancer in a well-defined French population: 1976–1995. J Hepatol 1998;29(5):802–6.
[26] McGlynn KA, Tsao L, Hsing AW, et al. International trends and patterns of primary liver cancer. Int J Cancer 2001;94:290–6.
[27] Taylor-Robinson SD, Foster GR, Arora S, et al. Increase in primary liver cancer in the UK, 1979–94. Lancet 1997;350(9085):1142–3.
[28] Okuda K, Fujimoto I, Hanai A, et al. Changing incidence of hepatocellular carcinoma in Japan. Cancer Res 1987;47(18):4967–72.

[29] El-Serag HB, Mason AC. Rising incidence of hepatocellular carcinoma in the United States. N Engl J Med 1999;340:745–50.
[30] El Serag HB, Davila JA, Petersen NJ, et al. The continuing increase in the incidence of hepatocellular carcinoma in the United States: an update. Ann Intern Med 2003;139(10): 817–23.
[31] Khan SA, Taylor-Robinson SD, Toledano MB, et al. Changing international trends in mortalitty rates for liver, biliary and pancreatic tumours. J Hepatol 2002;37(6):806–13.
[32] Levi F, Lucchini F, Negri E, et al. Cancer mortality in Europe, 1995–1999, and overview of trends since 1960. Int J Cancer 2004;110:155–69.
[33] Patel T. Increasing incidence and mortality of primary intrahepatic cholangiocarcinoma in the United States. Hepatology 2001;33(6):1353–7.
[34] Ribes J, Cleries R, Borras J, et al. Time trends in incidence and mortality for chronic liver disease and liver cancer in the interval 1980–1997 in Catalonia, Spain. Eur J Gastroenterol Hepatol 2004;16(9):865–72.
[35] Prince AM, Alcabes P. The risk of development of hepatocellular carcinoma in hepatitis B virus carrier in New York. A preliminary estimate using death-records matching. Hepatology 1982;2: 15–20.
[36] Dodd RY, Nath N. Increased risk for lethal forms of liver disease among HBsAg-positive blood donors in the United States. J Virol Methods 1987;17:81–94.
[37] Hall AJ, Winter PD, Wright R. Mortality of hepatitis B positive blood donors in England and Wales. Lancet 1985;1(8420):91–3.
[38] Crook PD, Jones ME, Hall AJ. Mortality of hepatitis B surface antigen-positive blood donors in England and Wales. Int J Epidemiol 2003;32:118–24.
[39] Oshima A, Tsukuma H, Hiyama T, et al. Follow-up study of HBsAg-positive blood donors with special reference to effect of drinking and smoking on development of liver cancer. Int J Cancer 1984;34:775–9.
[40] Sakuma K, Saitoh N, Kasai M, et al. Relative risks of death due to liver disease among Japanese male adults having various statuses for hepatitis B s and e antigen/antibody in serum: a prospective study. Hepatology 1988;8(6):1642–6.
[41] Sakuma K, Takahara T, Okuda K, et al. Prognosis of hepatitis B virus surface antigen carriers in relation to routine liver function tests: a prospective study. Gastroenterology 1982;83:114–7.
[42] Iijima T, Saitoh N, Nobutomo K, et al. A prospective cohort study of hepatitis B surface antigen carriers in a working population. Gann 1984;75:571–3.
[43] Tokudome S, Ikeda M, Matsushita K, et al. Hepatocellular carcinoma among female japanese hepatitis b virus carriers. Hepatogastroenterol 1987;34:246–8.
[44] Tokudome S, Ikeda M, Matsushita K, et al. Hepatocellular carcinoma among HBsAg positive blood donors in Fukuoka, Japan. Eur J Cancer Clin Oncol 1988;2:235–9.
[45] Beasley RP, Hwang LY, Lin CC, et al. Hepatocellular carcinoma and hepatitis B virus: a prospective study of 22707 men in Taiwan. Lancet 1981;ii:1129–33.
[46] Beasley RP. Hepatitis B virus. The major etiology of hepatocellular carcinoma. Cancer 1988; 61:1942–56.
[47] Yang H-I, Lu S-N, Liaw Y-F, et al. Hepatitis B e antigen and the risk of hepatocellular carcinoma. N Engl J Med 2002;347(3):168–74.
[48] Tu JT, Gao RN, Zhang DH, et al. Hepatitis B virus and primary liver cancer on Chongming Island, People's Republic of China. J Natl Cancer Inst Monogr 1985;69:213–5.
[49] Yeh FS, Yu MC, Mo CC, et al. Hepatitis B virus, Aflatoxins, and hepatocellular carcinoma in Southern Guangxi, China. Cancer Res 1989;49:2506–9.
[50] Ross RK, Yuan JM, Yu MC, et al. Urinary aflatoxin biomarkers and risk of hepatocellular carcinoma. Lancet 1992;339(8799):943–6.
[51] Evans AA, Chen G, Ross EA, et al. Eight-year follow-up of the 90,000-person Haimen City cohort: I. Hepatocellular carcinoma mortality, risk factors, and gender differences. Cancer Epidemiol Biomarkers Prev 2002;11(4):369–76.
[52] Alter MJ. Epidemiology and prevention of hepatitis B. Semin Liver Dis 2003;23(1):39–46.

[53] Evans AA, O'Connell AP, Pugh JC, et al. Geographic variations in viral load among Hepatitis B carriers with differing risks of hepatocellular carcinoma. Cancer Epidemiol Biomark Prev 1998; 7:559–65.
[54] Tang B, Kruger WD, Chen G, et al. Hepatitis B viremia is associated with increased risk of hepatocellular carcinoma in chronic carriers. J Med Virol 2004;72(1):35–40.
[55] Fattovich G. Natural history and prognosis of hepatitis B. Semin Liver Dis 2003;23(1):47–58.
[56] Abdel-Aziz F, Habib M, Mohamed MK, et al. Hepatitis C virus (HCV) infection in a community in the Nile Delta: population description and HCV prevalence. Hepatology 2000;32(1):111–5.
[57] Yoshizawa H. Hepatocellular carcinoma associated with hepatitis C virus infection in Japan: projection to other countries in the foreseeable future. Oncology 2002;62(suppl 1):8–17.
[58] Okuda K. Hepatitis C virus and hepatocellular carcinoma. In: Tabor E, Di Bisceglie AM, Purcell RH, editors. Etiology, pathology, and treatment of hepatocellular carcinoma in North America. Houston: PPC Gulf Publishing Company; 1991. p. 119–26.
[59] Wasley A, Alter MJ. Epidemiology of hepatitis C: geographic differences and temporal trends. Semin Liver Dis 2000;20:1–16.
[60] Frank C, Mohamed MK, Strickland GT, et al. The role of parenteral antischistosomal therapy in the spread of hepatitis C virus in Egypt. Lancet 2000;355(9207):887–91.
[61] Okuda K. Hepatitis C and hepatocellular carcinoma. In: Okuda K, Tabor E, editors. Liver cancer. New York: Churchill Livingstone (Elsevier); 1997. p. 39–50.
[62] El-Serag HB, Mason AC. Risk factors for the rising rates of primary liver cancer in the United States. Arch Intern Med 2000;160:3227–30.
[63] Bosch FX, Ribes J. The epidemiology of primary liver cancer: global epidemiology. In: Tabor E, editor. Viruses and liver cancer. New York: Elsevier Science; 2002. p. 1–16.
[64] Brechot C, Thiers V, Kremsdorf D, et al. Persistent hepatitis B virus infection in subjects without hepatitis B surface antigen: clinically significant or purely "occult"? Hepatology 2001;34(1): 194–203.
[65] Brechot C, Jaffredo F, Lagorce D, et al. Impact of HBV, HCV and GBV-C/HGV on hepatocellular carcinomas in Europe: results of a European concerted action. J Hepatol 1998;29(2): 173–83.
[66] Donato F, Boffetta P, Puoti M. A meta-analysis of epidemiological studies on the combined effect of hepatitis B and C virus infections in causing hepatocellular carcinoma. Int J Cancer 1998;75(3):347–54.
[67] International Agency for Research on Cancer (IARC). IARC monographs of the evaluation of carcinogenic risk to humans. Vol. 59. Hepatitis viruses. Lyon: IARC Press; 1994.
[68] Kao JH, Chen PJ, Lai MY, et al. Basal core promoter mutations of hepatitis B virus increase the risk of hepatocellular carcinoma in hepatitis B carriers. Gastroenterology 2003;124(2): 327–34.
[69] Chu CJ, Keeffe EB, Han SH, et al. Prevalence of HBV precore/core promoter variants in the United States. Hepatology 2003;38(3):619–28.
[70] Henry SH, Bosch FX. Foodborne disease and mycotoxin epidemiology. In: Hui YH, Smith RA, Spoerke Jr DG, editors. Foodborne diseases handbook, Vol. 3: Plant toxicants. New York: Marcel Dekker, Inc.; 2000. p. 593–626.
[71] Di Bisceglie AM, Carithers Jr RL, Gores GJ. Hepatocellular carcinoma. Hepatology 1998;28(4): 1161–5.
[72] Donato F, Tagger A, Chiesa R, et al. Hepatitis B and C virus infection, alcohol drinking, and hepatocellular carcinoma: a case–control study in Italy. Brescia HCC study. Hepatology 1997; 26(3):579–84.
[73] Kuper H, Tzonou A, Kaklamani E, et al. Tobacco smoking, alcohol consumption and their interaction in the causation of hepatocellular carcinoma. Int J Cancer 2000;85(4):498–502.
[74] Wang LY, You SL, Lu SN, et al. Risk of hepatocellular carcinoma and habits of alcohol drinking, betel quid chewing and cigarette smoking: a cohort of 2416 HBsAg-seropositive and 9421 HBsAg-seronegative male residents in Taiwan. Cancer Causes Control 2003;14(3):241–50.
[75] Chen ZM, Liu BQ, Boreham J, et al. Smoking and liver cancer in China: case–control

comparison of 36,000 liver cancer deaths vs. 17,000 cirrhosis deaths. Int J Cancer 2003;107(1):106–12.

[76] La Vecchia C, Tavani A, Franceschi S, et al. Oral contraceptives and cancer. A review of the evidence. Drug Saf 1996;14(4):260–72.

[77] Kew MC, Song E, Mohammed A, et al. Contraceptive steroids as a risk factor for hepatocellular carcinoma: a case/control study in South African black women. Hepatology 1990;11(2):298–302.

[78] Mant JW, Vessey MP. Trends in mortality from primary liver cancer in England and Wales 1975–92: influence of oral contraceptives. Br J Cancer 1995;72(3):800–3.

[79] Waetjen LE, Grimes DA. Oral contraceptives and primary liver cancer: temporal trends in three countries. Obstet Gynecol 1996;88(6):945–9.

[80] Beral V, Hermon C, Kay C, et al. Mortality associated with oral contraceptive use: 25 year follow up of cohort of 46 000 women from Royal College of General Practitioners' oral contraception study. BMJ 1999;318(7176):96–100.

[81] The Collaborative MILTS Project Team. Oral contraceptives and liver cancer. Results of the Multicentre International Liver Tumor Study (MILTS). Contraception 1997;56(5):275–84.

[82] Yu MW, Chang HC, Chang SC, et al. Role of reproductive factors in hepatocellular carcinoma: impact on hepatitis B- and C-related risk. Hepatology 2003;38(6):1393–400.

[83] Lagiou P, Kuper H, Stuver SO, et al. Role of diabetes mellitus in the etiology of hepatocellular carcinoma. J Natl Cancer Inst 2000;92(13):1096–9.

[84] Wideroff L, Gridley G, Mellemkjaer L, et al. Cancer incidence in a population-based cohort of patients hospitalized with diabetes mellitus in Denmark. J Natl Cancer Inst 1997;89(18):1360–5.

[85] Adami HO, Chow WH, Nyren O, et al. Excess risk of primary liver cancer in patients with diabetes mellitus. J Natl Cancer Inst 1996;88(20):1472–7.

[86] El Serag HB, Tran T, Everhart JE. Diabetes increases the risk of chronic liver disease and hepatocellular carcinoma. Gastroenterology 2004;126(2):460–8.

[87] Sorensen HT, Mellemkjaer L, Jepsen P, et al. Risk of cancer in patients hospitalized with fatty liver: a Danish cohort study. J Clin Gastroenterol 2003;36(4):356–9.

[88] Whittle HC, Maine N, Pilkington J, et al. Long-term efficacy of continuing hepatitis B vaccination in infancy in two Gambian villages. Lancet 1995;345(8957):1089–92.

[89] Hsu HM, Chen DS, Chuang CH, et al. Efficacy of a mass hepatitis B vaccination program in Taiwan. Studies on 3464 infants of hepatitis B surface antigen-carrier mothers. JAMA 1988;260(15):2231–5.

[90] Chang MH, Chen CJ, Lai MS, et al. Universal hepatitis B vaccination in Taiwan and the incidence of hepatocellular carcinoma in children. Taiwan Childhood Hepatoma Study Group. N Engl J Med 1997;336(26):1855–9.

[91] Lee MS, Kim DH, Kim H, et al. Hepatitis B vaccination and reduced risk of primary liver cancer among male adults: a cohort study in Korea. Int J Epidemiol 1998;27(2):316–9.

[92] Tabor E, Yu MY, Hewlett I, et al. Summary of a workshop on the implementation of NAT to screen donors of blood and plasma for viruses. Transfusion 2000;40(10):1273–5.

ELSEVIER
SAUNDERS

Clin Liver Dis 9 (2005) 213–223

CLINICS IN
LIVER DISEASE

# Staging for Liver Cancer

Bruno Daniele, MD, PhD[a,*], Francesco Perrone, MD, PhD[b]

[a]*Medical Oncology Unit, "G. Rummo" Hospital, Benevento, Italy*
[b]*Clinical Trials Unit, National Cancer Institute, Napoli, Italy*

Both cancer staging systems and prognostic scores distinctly provide important information in clinical practice and research setting [1]. They can be used for decision making in individual patients and are useful to inform patients about their likely outcome (survival probability); in the assessment of treatment benefits from a homogeneous group of patients with respect to their expected outcome; in the combination of data from independent trials through meta-analyses. Finally, knowledge of the prognostic factors may assist in determining necessary sample size and the variables needed for stratified allocation in treatment trials. However, staging and prognostic systems meet different demands and are meant for different uses. Table 1 summarizes the different features of staging systems and prognostic scores.

## Cancer staging systems

Cancer staging systems consider only the extention of the disease. The TNM is the most widely used cancer staging system. It classifies solid tumors according to the anatomic extent before treatment and is based on the extent of primary tumor (T), presence of lymph node metastasis (N), and distant metastasis (M). There may be a clinical classification (cTNM) based on clinical or imaging findings and a pathologic classification (pTNM). Based on TNM, patients are eventually classified within a stage, that ranges from I to IV, each characterizing a different prognosis [2].

* Corresponding author.
*E-mail address:* bruno.daniele@ao-rummo.it (B. Daniele).

1089-3261/05/$ – see front matter 
doi:10.1016/j.cld.2004.12.003

***liver.theclinics.com***

Table 1
Differential characteristics of staging systems and prognostic scores in clinical oncology

| | Staging systems | Prognostic scores |
|---|---|---|
| Object | Extension of cancer. | All variables possibly affecting outcome (life expectancy), including staging. |
| Effect on treatment choice | Direct. | Indirect, through cost-benefit considerations. |
| Consideration of available treatment | Must be taken into account when developing and updating. Invasive procedures (diagnostic and therapeutic at the same time) can be integrated. | Can be ignored. Must be considered when there are well-established treatments, used worldwide with strong evidence of efficacy, and generalizable to the majority of patients. |
| Precision | Required. Must be checked. | In theory welcome, but it is hardly achieved. |
| Time and procedures | Better if short and simple. May be long, complicated, and require technology application. | Short and simple. |
| Invasive procedures | Acceptable, if needed. | Not acceptable behind those applied for staging. |
| Use of physician's subjective judgement | Acceptable only for clinical staging definition. | Not optimal because potentially biased |
| Use of patient's subjective judgement | Not acceptable. | Not optimal but acceptable, because its heterogeneity may refer to true patients variability. |
| Prognostic ability | Possible, but not necessary. | Required by definition. |
| Timing | Immediately after diagnosis. Pathologic staging may be defined after initial surgical treatment. | As for staging systems, but may be refined according to treatment effect. |

The staging systems are of great value when several different therapeutic approaches are available, and their application depends on the extention of the neoplastic disease. Indeed, surgery and radiotherapy produce local control of the disease and are optimally applied if the cancer is limited to the primary organ or to its regional nodes or close soft tissues. On the other hand, systemic treatments are needed for cancers at an advanced or metastatic stage. A further distinction of early-stage cancer within substages may guide the therapeutic choice among, for instance, aggressive or conservative surgery or among different types of locoregional treatment (eg, surgery, radiotherapy, or other tools for local ablation). Therefore, it is intuitive that staging systems for different cancers should be produced and verified in the light of the available therapeutic strategies, their technical requirements, and their evolution across time. The quality of staging systems is substantially based on their precision and efficiency in determining clear-cut indications for treatment decision making. In some cases, the diagnostic workup needed to obtain a precise definition of tumor extension can be heavy and time consuming, depending on how important the assignment of patients to one or another category of the staging system is for the treatment strategy. Invasive procedures (including surgery or arteriography) can be required to optimally define stage. Generally, staging systems precisely define extention because they are mostly based on objective measures of tumor size, although they share the limitations of the diagnostic tools employed. To be fully implemented, a cancer staging system must be validated and reproducible. This means that it can be translated on an international basis, and that the staging procedures should not be too complex and the interpretation of their results too subjective. Because the extent of the cancer and its impact on treatment outcome are commonly the strongest determinants of patients survival, staging systems are frequently, but not always, also able to predict prognosis.

## Prognostic scores

Prognostic scores should take into account all variables eventually affecting the survival of patients, including, but not limited to, the extension of cancer. Additional variables may include the characteristics of patients (sex, age, race), the assessment of general health status and performance status, concomitant diseases, and the biologic characteristics of the cancer (eg, histology, grade of differentiation, molecular markers). For many cancers there is a number of established prognostic factors that do not directly measure disease extension, and a lot of studies are carried on to identify new factors. The primary aim of a prognostic score is to produce a reasonable estimation of life expectancy. Although driving treatment choice cannot be considered the primary aim of a prognostic score, the knowledge of the expected survival may have consequences on treatment decision making, particularly when a cost–benefit analysis has to be done, weighting pros and cons of the available treatment procedures. Contrary to staging systems that can require heavy and time-consuming procedures, prognostic scores should be easy to calculate, although this can translate, of course, in a lower precision. However, strategies can be implemented to keep the reduced precision within reasonable limits. Factors that can be only subjectively assessed by the physicians should be avoided or their use minimized, because they can be systematically biased by personal inclination. In contrast, subjective assessments made by the patients can be taken into account because their unpredictable variability does ultimately refer to the true heterogeneity of individual patients.

A prognostic score should be calculated after the staging procedures are done and, obviously, it must take into account the stage classification. When all the prognostic information needed to build the score is available before any treatment is performed, the prognostic score can be calculated before treatment, and its survival prediction can somehow affect the treatment decision. There are instances, however, like early breast cancer, where the information derived from the pathologic examination of surgically removed specimens are necessary to calculate the score. In these cases, a prognostic score can be useful both to drive the choice of additional treatments (eg, adjuvant treatment) and to define the follow-up schedules according to the perceived risk of relapse or death. The identification and use of prognostic scores to be assessed after an initial treatment (mostly surgical) of cancer seems reasonable only if some requirements are satisfied: (1) there is a general agreement on the initial therapeutic approach; (2) the efficacy of such approach is demonstrated with a high level of evidence; (3) and the proportion of patients with the disease who are candidates for this approach is high. If such requirements are not met (eg, no agreement on initial treatment approach, lack of reliable randomized trials testing the efficacy of treatments, and so on) a prognostic score needs to be assessed before any treatment is given, and only large validation studies can deal with the performance of the score within subgroups of patients treated homogeneously.

## The construction of a prognostic score

Table 2 summarizes some of the requirements for the construction of a prognostic score. Prognostic scores can be built by applying an appropriate methodology. First, a database is required including all established prognostic factors as well as treatment and outcome information for all patients. The database should be sufficiently large and possibly multicentric, to be representative of several settings and not biased by procedures that could be typical of one

Table 2
Requirements for the construction of a prognostic score

| | |
|---|---|
| Base of data | |
| Size | The larger the better. |
| Source | Multicenter better than single institution, to account for heterogeneity and improve generalizability. |
| | Clinical practice better than clinical trials, because selection criteria may reduce generalizability. |
| Collection | Prospective: optimal but inefficient. |
| | Retrospective: suboptimal but efficient. |
| Variables | All known prognostic factors, excluding those still considered as experimental, and all known previous scores. |
| Analysis | |
| Internal validity | Appropriate statistical tests, including multivariable models. |
| | Splitting of data set into training and testing samples to reduce overfitting phenomenon. |
| | Comparison with other available prognostic scores through adequate statistical methods. |
| External validity | Validation in data set differing from the initial data base because of: |
| | type of hospital |
| | geographic location |
| | race |
| | epidemiologic characteristics (eg, risk or etiologic factors) |

single center and not reproducible outside of it. Patients included in the database should be treated and followed according to widely accepted strategies, as much as possible coherent with common clinical practice. The database can be collected prospectively for prognostic studies (this strategy requires time and is not efficient) or could be retrospective, either resulting from previously conducted clinical trials (in this case, the enrolment criteria of the trials can reduce the generalizability of the prognostic findings) or built by retrospectively collecting data from unselected series of patients (eg, all the patients seen in a predefined time window). The last option is probably the most efficient, but because of its retrospective nature it is subject to the typical selection bias of retrospective data collection and to the problem of the missing data that can make the results unreliable. Some strategies can, however, be implemented to improve the reliability of the retrospective prognostic analysis; if the database is sufficiently large, it can be divided in a training sample (where analyses are conducted to identify the optimal way to predict prognosis) and one or more testing samples (eventually created by random procedures) to test the proposed tool, reducing the risk of overfitting. Appropriate statistical methods should be applied to identify the optimal combination of prognostic factors that can be used to calculate an index. Multivariable analysis should be applied, which can also produce estimates of the relative weight that each variable can have in the index. The proposed index should be compared with those already available, and the relative merits should be appropriately studied both in terms of statistical methods and in terms of clinical applicability and generalizability. Finally, independent validation is required to prove the external validity of the score, which should be tested for feasibility (manoeuvrability of the scoring system, ease of data identification, and so on), generalizability (in different geographic areas, in different hospital settings, and so on), and validity compared with other previously available prognostic scores.

## Issues of staging and prognosis in hepatocellular carcinoma

Based on the previous concepts, hepatocellular carcinoma (HCC) is a case in which:

- prognostic scores are absolutely required because the patient outcome largely depends upon variables other than tumor extension (ie, concomitant liver disease)
- the optimal time for identification and application of prognostic scores is before giving any treatment because: (a) there is no agreement on what is the optimal treatment for almost all the stages of the disease; (b) there is no solid evidence of efficacy of any available treatment coming from well conducted randomized trials; (c) there is no treatment sufficiently universal and widely used to be proposed to the majority of patients.

## Prognosis of hepatocellular carcinoma

HCC most often develops in cirrhotic patients, with a variable degree of liver failure [3]. Therefore, the prognosis of HCC patients is dictated by both cancer diffusion and residual liver function. This explains why staging systems that take into account only liver function (Child-Pugh) or tumor extent (TNM) do not perform well in these patients [4,5]. An attempt to combine liver function and tumor extent was first made by Okuda [6], who grouped HCC patients within three stages depending on tumor volume, presence of ascites, and concentration of bilirubin and albumin. The Okuda staging system for HCC was widely used for 2 decades. During the 1990s, the availability of more sophisticated imaging techniques for diagnosis and the implementation of screening programs to detect early HCC in cirrhotic patients led to the diagnosis of very small HCCs in contrast to the often symptomatic disease at diagnosis when Okuda introduced his staging system. In addition, a number of individual findings (eg, vascular invasion) had been credited with prognostic values during the past years. Thus, several prognostic scores, including several factors, have been proposed worldwide (Table 3).

Table 3
Factors including in prognostic scores for hepatocellular carcinoma

| Prognostic score | Assessment of liver function | Assessment of tumor extention | Assessment of vascular invasion | Other |
|---|---|---|---|---|
| AJCC sTNM | | Number and size of nodules | Portal obstruction<br>Microvascular invasion | Grade of liver fibrosis |
| BCLC | Child-Pugh<br>Serum bilirubin<br>Portal pressure | Number and size of nodules | | Performance status<br>Associated diseases<br>Okuda stage |
| CLIP | Child-Pugh | Number and volume of nodules | Portal obstruction | Serum alpha-fetoprotein value |
| CUPI | Serum bilirubin | TNM stage | | Symptoms<br>Serum alpha-fetoprotein value<br>Serum alkaline phosfatase<br>Ascites |
| GRECH | Serum bilirubin | | Portal obstruction | Serum alkaline phosfatase<br>Serum alpha-fetoprotein<br>Performance status |
| VISUM | Serum bilirubin<br>Prothrombin time | Volume of nodules<br>Enlarged lymph nodes | Portal obstruction | Serum alpha-fetoprotein |

*Abbreviations:* AJCC, American Joint Commission on Cancer; BCLC, Barcelona Clinic Liver Cancer; CLIP, Cancer of the Liver Italian Program; CUPI, Chinese University Prognostic Index; GRECH, Groupe d'Etude et de Traitement du Carcinome Hepatocellulaire; VISUM, Vienna Survival Model.

## The American Joint Commission on Cancer/TNM system

In the past years, it has become clear that the inclusion of some non anatomic factors to the classic TNM system is necessary to estimate optimally prognosis. Non anatomic factors include histologic type and age in thyroid carcinoma; high grade in bone and soft tissue tumors and prostate cancer; serum tumor markers in testicular cancer, PSA in prostate cancer [2].

Therefore, a new simplified classification for HCC patients, called sTNM, including non anatomic factors such as liver fibrosis or microvascular invasion, was developed using a database of 591 patients who underwent complete resection of HCC between 1980 and 1998 at four centers [7]. Because the cohort studied included only patients who had a liver resection, and because this system requires an assessment of the degree of liver fibrosis as well as microvascular invasion, the application of the sTNM is limited to patients who had a liver resection. In addition, patients presenting with HCC who are amenable to surgical resection represent a minority of the whole population of HCC patients. The sTNM has not been validated prospectively.

## The Barcelona Clinic Liver Cancer staging classification

The Barcelona Clinic Liver Cancer (BCLC) staging classification [8] represents an a priori stratification of HCC patients into four major categories (early, intemediate, advanced, and terminal stage). Based on the attribution of the patients to one of these categories, specific treatments are indicated. The BCLC includes the assessment of patient performance status, which is not an objective measurement. In addition, the measurement of portal pressure, one of the parameters included in the classification, may be complex and not precise. The BCLC classification has not been validated either prospectively or externally.

## The Cancer of the Liver Italian Group score

The Cancer of the Liver Italian Program (CLIP) developed a new HCC staging system—the CLIP score—using a methodologically appropriate procedure. The first study was retrospective [9]: in a population of HCC patients, univariate analysis was used to select individual findings with prognostic value to be included in a multivariate analysis. Then, the Cox model was applied to select variables for the final model, always using locoregional treatment as a stratification factor. An internal crossvalidation procedure was applied, splitting the whole sample in a training (67%) and in a testing sample (33%). A simple scoring system (Table 4) was derived assigning linear scores (0, 1 or 2) to the covariates of the final model: the higher the final score, the worse the prognosis. The prognostic validity of the CLIP score was assessed on 10 testing samples. The second step was the validation of the CLIP score in an independent group of

Table 4
CLIP scoring system

| | Scoring | | |
|---|---|---|---|
| Variables | 0 | 1 | 2 |
| Child-Pugh stage | A | B | C |
| Tumor morphology | Uninodular and extention $\leq 50\%$ | Multinodular and extention $\leq 50\%$ | Massive or extention $> 50\%$ |
| AFP (ng/mL) | $< 400$ | $\geq 400$ | |
| Portal vein thrombosis | No | Yes | |

*Abbreviations:* AFP, alpha-fetoprotein; CLIP, Cancer of the Liver Italian Program.

patients prospectively enrolled [10]. The study showed that, compared with the Okuda staging system, the CLIP score gives more precise prognostic information, is statistically more efficient, and has a greater predictive power on survival. Finally, the CLIP score has been externally validated (Table 5). Recently, the American Hepato-Pancreatic-Biliary Association/American Joint Commission on Cancer Consensus Conference on Staging of Hepatocellular Carcinoma recommended the CLIP system as the primary clinical staging that can be applied to all patients [11]. As it has been said in a comment on the Consensus Statement [12], "all new clinical trials and clinical descriptions of HCC should include categorization by CLIP score." However, the CLIP system may need to be adapted to different situations. In Western countries, where early detection of HCC is more frequent, the highest CLIP categories (4 to 6 or 3 to 6) should be considered together because they comprise small numbers of patients that may show an erratic behavior. For the same reason, in countries where the expected survival is very short, the lower CLIP categories (0 to 2) should be considered together.

## The Chinese University Prognostic Index

Survival of HCC patients appears to be different according to their racial origin. The shorter survival of Asian patients may be due to the different etiology of the disease, mainly Hepatitis B virus (HBV), or more severe underlying liver disease. Based on the above observations, a research group in Hong Kong

Table 5
Studies of external validation of the CLIP score

| Author | Number of patients | Population | Type of study |
|---|---|---|---|
| Farinati [17] | 154 | Italian | Prospective |
| Ueno [18] | 662 | Japanese | Retrospective |
| Leung [13] | 926 | Chinese | Prospective |
| Zhao [19] | 174 | Chinese | Retrospective |
| Sherman [20] | 257 | Canadian | Retrospective |
| Kudo [21] | 722 | Japanese | Retrospective |

*Abbreviation:* CLIP, Cancer of the Liver Italian Program.

developed the Chinese University Prognostic Index (CUPI), assessing the value of independent prognostic variables from a database of 926 adult Chinese patients with HCC observed in a single center in Hong Kong from 1996 to 1998 [13]. Some baseline and outcome characteristics of this group of patients indicate that they are not representative of the HCC profile typically seen in Western countries or in Japan. For instance, the majority (79%) of HCCs was HBV-related, while only 3% was related to Hepatitis C virus (HCV). In addition, about 60% of patients received only supportive care and survival was extremely short (median of 19 weeks, 23% at 1 year, and only 6% at 2 years). The study sample was split randomly in two sets: a training set (75% of the population) and a confirmatory set (25% of the population). The analysis identified alpha-fetoprotein, total bilirubin, alkaline phosphatase, ascites, and asymptomatic disease on presentation as independent prognostic variables that were added to the TNM stage. Vascular invasion was not included among the variables. Different scores were assigned to each variable, and three groups of patients with a different survival were identified. The CUPI score appeared more discriminative than the TNM alone, the Okuda and the CLIP score. In the case of CLIP score, however, discrimination was poor only for patients with a low score (ie, those with an expected better prognosis), which represented only 6% of the whole population. In view of this, comparing CLIP and CUPI scores in this population may have led to misleading conclusions. The CUPI score has not been prospectively validated.

## The Groupe d'Etude et de Traitement du Carcinome Hepatocellulaire score

The Groupe d'Etude et de Traitement du Carcinome Hepatocellulaire (GRECH) score was developed using data from 779 HCC patients prospectively recruited in 24 participating centers in France, Belgium, and Canada from 1990 to 1992 [14]. An appropriate methodology was used by developing the score in a training sample and then validating it in a testing sample. The classification distinguishes three groups of patients associated with different estimated risk of death. This score includes the assessment of patient performance status, which is not an objective measurement. The GRECH score has not been externally validated.

## The Vienna Survival Model

The Vienna Survival Model (VISUM) score is a prognostic model developed from baseline data obtained by 245 consecutive HCC patients seen in a single Austrian Institution from 1991 to 1998, and then tested on an independent group of 89 patients, seen from April 1998 to September 1999 [15]. In these patients, HCC was diagnosed mainly at an advanced stage. The VISUM score included serum bilirubin, serum alpha-fetoprotein, prothrombin time, tumor volume, enlarged lymph nodes, portal vein thrombosis, and separated three prognostic stages with different median survival. The VISUM score has not been prospectively validated.

## Evolution of the prognostic scores

The construction of a prognostic score is a dynamic process, due to the emerging value of biologic, genetic, and molecular factors in the staging of various carcinomas, including HCC, as well as to the trend toward individualized therapy. It remains crucial, however, that the methodology of assessment of independent prognostic factors is appropriate. Specifically, to incorporate a new prognostic factor in any other cancer prognostic system a significant influence on prognosis independent of the prognostic system must be proven.

In the case of HCC, an attempt was made to include some serum markers credited with prognostic value in individual studies (sICAM, sIL2-R, p53Ab, and so on) into the CLIP score [16]. Unfortunately, the prognostic value of the single variables was lost when included in the CLIP score, further underlying the need for an appropriate methodologic approach to the development of cancer prognostic systems.

## Summary

Cancer prognostic systems are essential for designing and conducting clinical trials, assessing the impact of new technologies, and comparing different patient populations. The development of a cancer prognostic system should be considered a dynamic process, as the system needs to be periodically updated when new prognostic factors become available. It is important that changes to cancer prognostic systems follow an appropriate methodology. A prognostic system for patients with HCC needs to combine tumor extent and residual liver function. At the moment, the CLIP score, which is easy to calculate and based on objective parameters, has been validated prospectively and in different populations represents the most useful prognostic system for HCC.

## References

[1] Kavanagh JJ. Principles of diagnosis and staging. In: Fisch MJ, Bruera E, editors. Handbook of advanced cancer care. Cambridge: Cambridge University Press; 2003. p. 3–11.

[2] Yarbro JW, Page DL, Fielding LP, et al. American Joint Committee on Cancer prognostic factors consensus conference. Cancer 1999;86(11):2436–46.

[3] Fattovich G, Stroffolini T, Aagni I, et al. Hepatocellular carcinoma in cirrhosis. Incidence and risk factors. Gastroenterology 2004;127(5 Suppl. 2):S35–50.

[4] Izumi R, Shimizu K, Ii T, et al. Prognostic factors of hepatocellular carcinoma in patients undergoing hepatic resection. Gastroenterology 1994;106(3):720–7.

[5] Llovet JM, Bruix J, Fuster J, et al. Liver transplantation for small hepatocellular carcinoma: the tumor-node-metastasis classification deos not have prognostic power. Hepatology 1998;27(6): 1572–7.
[6] Okuda K, Ohtsuki T, Obata H, et al. Natural history of hepatocellular carcinoma and prognosis in relation to treatment. Study of 850 patients. Cancer 1985;56(4):918–28.
[7] Vauthey JN, Lauwers GY, Esnaola NF, et al. Simplified staging for hepatocellular carcinoma. J Clin Oncol 2002;20(6):1527–36.
[8] Llovet JM, Bru C, Bruix J. Prognosis of hepatocellular carcinoma: the BCLC staging classification. Semin Liver Dis 1999;19(3):329–38.
[9] The Cancer of the Liver Italian Program (CLIP) Investigators. A new prognostic system for hepatocellular carcinoma: a retrospective study of 435 patients. Hepatology 1998;28(3):751–5.
[10] The Cancer of the Liver Italian Program (CLIP) Investigators. Prospective validation of the CLIP score: a new prognostic system for patients with cirrhosis and hepatocellular carcinoma. Hepatology 2000;31(4):840–5.
[11] Henderson JM, Sherman M, Tavill A, et al. AHPBA/AJCC Consensus Conference on Staging of Hepatocellular Carcinoma: consensus statement. HPB 2003;5(4):243–50.
[12] Di Bisceglie AM, Strasberg S. A common staging system for hepatocellular carcinoma. Hepatology 2004;39(2):550–1.
[13] Leung TWT, Tang AMY, Zee B, et al. Construction of the Chinese University prognostic index for hepatocellular carcinoma and comparison with the TNM staging system, the Okuda staging system and the Cancer of the Liver Italian Program staging system. Cancer 2002; 94(6):1760–9.
[14] Chevret S, Trinchet JC, Mathieu D, et al. A new prognostic classification for predicting survival in patients with hepatocellular carcinoma. Groupe d'Etude et de Traitement du Carcinome Hepatocellulaire. J Hepatol 1999;31(1):133–41.
[15] Schoniger-Hekele M, Muller C, Kutilek M, et al. Hepatocellular carcinoma in central Europe: prognostic features and survival. Gut 2001;48(1):103–9.
[16] Parasole R, Izzo F, Perrone F, et al. Prognostic value of serum biological markers in patients with hepatocellular carcinoma. Clin Cancer Res 2001;7(11):3504–9.
[17] Farinati F, Rinaldi M, Gianni S, et al. How should patients with hepatocellular carcinoma be staged? Validation of a new prognostic system. Cancer 2000;89(11):2266–73.
[18] Ueno S, Tanabe G, Sako K, et al. Discrimination value of the new prognostic system (CLIP score) for hepatocellular carcinoma in 662 Japanese Patients. Hepatology 2001;34(3):529–34.
[19] Zhao WH, Ma ZM, Zhou XR, et al. Prediction of recurrence and prognosis in patients with hepatocellular carcinoma after resection by use of CLIP score. World J Gastroenterol 2002; 8(2):237–42.
[20] Levy I, Sherman M. Staging of hepatocellular carcinoma: assessment of the CLIP, Okuda, and Child-Pugh staging systems in a cohort of 257 patients in Toronto. Gut 2002;50(6):881–5.
[21] Kudo M, Chung H, Osaki Y. Prognostic staging system for hepatocellular carcinoma (CLIP score): its value and limitations, and a proposal for a new staging system, the Japan Integrated Staging Score (JIS score). J Gastroenterol 2003;38(3):207–15.

ELSEVIER
SAUNDERS

Clin Liver Dis 9 (2005) 225–234

CLINICS IN
LIVER DISEASE

# The Use of Decision Analytic Models to Inform Clinical Decision Making in the Management of Hepatocellular Carcinoma

W. Ray Kim, MD, MBA

*Mayo Clinic College of Medicine, Division of Gastroenterology, Mayo Building, East 16, 200 Fist Street SW, Rochester, MN 55905, USA*

Clinical decision making commonly involves selection among two or more alternatives, all of which entail varying degrees of uncertainty about the consequences that will follow that decision. Medical decision analysis is a quantitative tool to help evaluate outcome of possible strategies in the diagnosis and management of diseases, while taking into account uncertainty about the results of the selected strategies [1]. Uncertainty derives from a host of factors such as imperfections in diagnostic testing, variability in the natural history of disease, and the random nature of treatment response and complications, apart from what may be predicted from patient-specific factors or comorbid conditions. Using decision analysis, decision makers try to optimize the expected outcome of a decision, incorporating the probabilistic nature of this uncertainty [2].

## Decision tree analysis

The simplest form of decision analysis is the decision tree. Fig. 1 demonstrates a simple decision tree that illustrates what may be entailed in the decision whether to perform screening for hepatocellular carcinoma (HCC) in patients with cirrhosis. From the initial stem of the tree, referred to as the decision node (represented by a square by convention), two or more branches of the tree originate, which represent different strategies (Fig. 1). Each branch may result in one

This work was supported by NIH Grant DK 60617.
*E-mail address:* kim.woong@mayo.edu


doi:10.1016/j.cld.2004.12.004

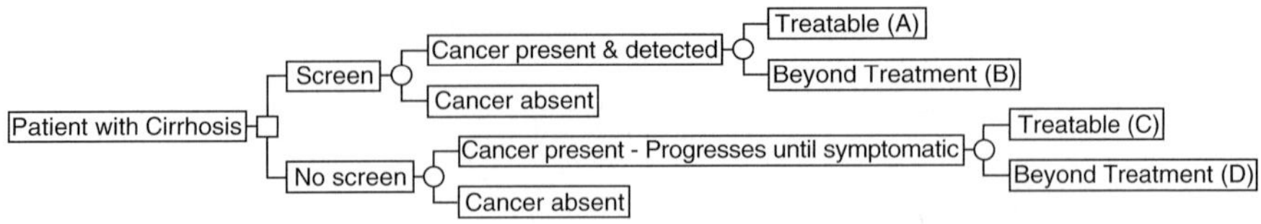


Fig. 1. A simple decision tree describing the decision and potential consequences of screening for HCC.

or more outcomes, shown as subsequent secondary branches. At each branching point (referred to as a chance node, represented by circles), the probability of each subsequent event dictates likelihood for individual outcomes to materialize.

In the example illustrated in Fig. 1, the clinician is faced with a decision whether to screen a patient with liver cirrhosis for HCC. The first strategy, screening, results in early detection of HCC before it becomes symptomatic. Because of the early detection, there is a high likelihood that the tumor is treatable, leading to a successful outcome. In the case where a cancer is absent, the screening will inform the clinician accordingly. In the second strategy in which no screening is performed, HCC will not be detected until it becomes symptomatic, which will trigger a diagnostic cascade eventually to reveal that the chance for a successful outcome is smaller than when the screening is instituted.

Eventual outcomes in a decision tree are the terminal branches of the model, and can be life, death, morbidity, or any other state of health or disease. In this simplified example, the most direct outcome of interest is the probability of detecting cancers at a treatable stage, which presumably will lead to extension of life or avoidance of death. In other words, in Fig. 1, the probability of outcome (A) is greater than outcome (C) and that of outcome (B) is smaller than outcome (D).

Once the decision–outcome relationship is identified and a tree is constructed accordingly, numerical data input may be used to derive rational conclusions from the model. This is accomplished through "folding back" of the tree, which is a series of expected value calculations. The expected value at a node is the sum of all products of probabilities and outcomes distal to that node. These calculations start on the right side of the tree and progress to the left toward the decision node.

Let us consider a numerical example. Fig. 2 represents the same decision tree as shown in Fig. 1, except that it shows numerical data about probabilities and

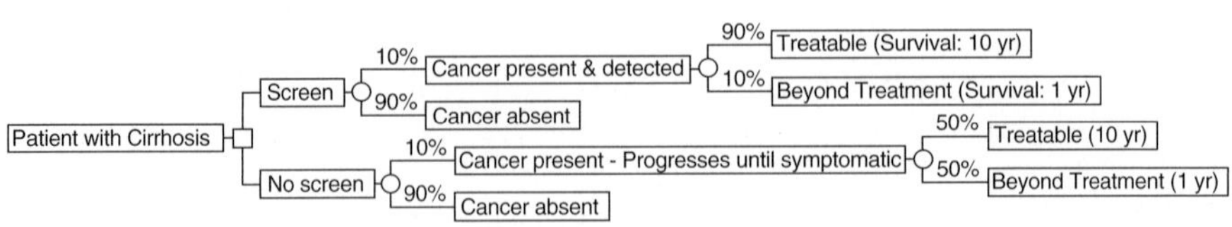


Fig. 2. A simple decision tree describing the decision and potential consequences of screening for HCC.

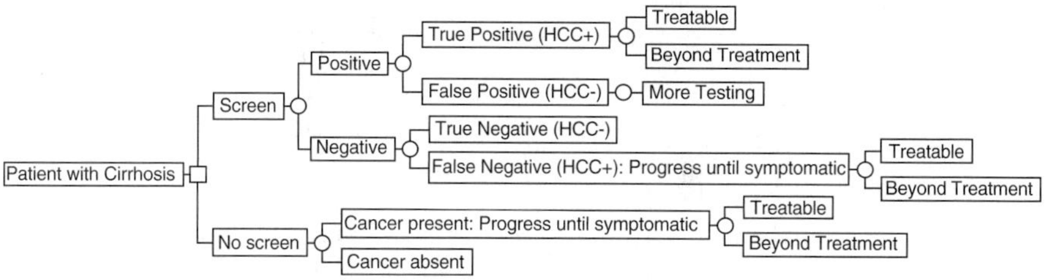


Fig. 3. A decision tree incorporating diagnostic characteristics of the screening test. Sensitivity and specificity of the test determines the proportions of true and false positives and negatives.

outcomes. If, hypothetically, there is a 10% probability that HCC is present and all of them will be detected by screening, those who undergo screening will have a 90% chance to be treatable, leading to 10 years of survival. In the remaining 10%, HCC is beyond treatment and only allows 1 year of survival. Based on these data, the expected survival of a patient who underwent screening and was detected to have HCC is 4.6 years (90% × 5 years + 10% × 1 year). Based on 10% prevalence of HCC, the expected survival of all patients undergoing screening is 9.46 years (10% × 4.6 years + 90% × 10 years). On the other hand, if screening was not performed, the expected survival of those who develop HCC is 3 years (50% × 5 years + 50% × 1 year). The expected survival of those who do not undergo screening is 9.3 years (10% × 3 years + 90% × 10 years). Thus, in this simplified example, screening is associated with a gain of 0.16 (9.46–9.3) years, or slightly less than 2 months, in survival.

Although the example shown in Figs. 1 and 2 helps describing the pros and cons associated with screening, most readers will immediately recognize that this is an oversimplification of the real-world counterpart. For one thing, it assumes that whatever screening modality is used, it is able to detect HCC that is present without an error. In real life, no screening or diagnostic tests are perfect. Sensitivity of a test refers to the proportion of positive results out of all cases with disease, whereas specificity is the proportion of negative results among those without disease. As shown in Fig. 3, a test with sensitivity less than 100% leads to negative results in some cases with disease (false negatives). Imperfect specificity leads to false positive results in cases without disease. Incorporating these considerations to the decision tree renders it noticeably more complicated. Although this still is oversimplification of the real situation (see the next section), this example illustrates how a simple tree can be expanded to incorporate more complicated scenarios in decision analyses and explicitly deal with uncertainties.

## Markov models

Although the analysis illustrated in Fig. 3 is a more realistic improvement over that in Fig. 1, it nevertheless is still too simplistic in that it is not able take into account the repetitive nature of screening. Obviously, performing a screening test

Fig. 4. A simple two-stage Markov model representing transition of patients from cirrhosis to HCC stages.

only once in patients with cirrhosis who are at a continual risk of developing HCC does not make much sense. To be able to incorporate the time dimension, the analyst may use a Markov model, a common technique to model the natural history of a disease in decision analysis [3]. In Markov models, a disease process is modeled as a series of health states, in and out of which patients move over time.

Fig. 4 represents a simple Markov model that depicts transition of patients with cirrhosis to HCC. Thus, a Markov model consists of health (or disease) states and transitions. In this example, both cirrhosis and HCC are disease states, and there is a simple transition from the former to the latter. For this model to be informative, the analyst needs to be able to assess the rate at which this transition occurs. This rate is defined by the length of time of observation and probability with which the transition occurs with that period of observation.

In generic terms, Markov models are composed of the following four elements.

1. Health states: discrete health (or disease) states that describe stages in the natural history of a disease.
2. Transition: movement of patients into and out of health states.
3. Defined unit of time: the length of time for each cycle of transition to occur.
4. Transition probabilities: the probabilities with which transitions occur between health states over unit of time.

As with decision tree analyses, numerical data are necessary to quantitatively implement Markov models. For example, Degos et al reported that the annual incidence of HCC among patients with compensated liver cirrhosis (ie, transition probability from cirrhosis to HCC over 1 year) was 2.6% [4]. In Table 1, we create a cohort of 1000 (an arbitrary round number) individuals with compensated cirrhosis. At time zero all members of the cohort have compensated cirrhosis with no HCC. If we choose the length of the cycle to be 1 year, during

Table 1
A simple two-stage Markov model describing transitions from cirrhosis to HCC

| Year | Cirrhosis | HCC |
|---|---|---|
| Zero | 1000 | 0 |
| 1 | 974 | 26 |
| 2 | 949 | 51 |
| — | — | — |
| 10 | 768 | 232 |
| 20 | 590 | 410 |
| 30 | 454 | 546 |

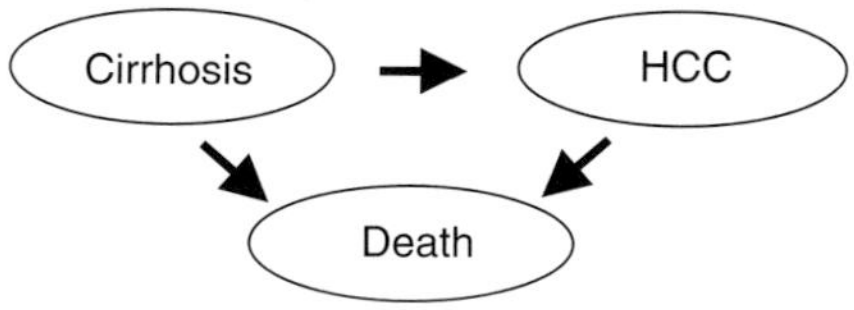


Fig. 5. A simple three-stage Markov model representing transition of patients from cirrhosis to HCC, HCC to death, cirrhosis to death.

the first cycle, 2.6% of the cohort will have developed HCC. Thus, at the end of the first year, there are 26 with HCC.

During the second year, another 2.6% of the remaining 974 with cirrhosis will develop HCC (974 × 2.6% = 25). Thus, by the end of the second year, there are 51 (26 + 25) with HCC. This process may be repeated over many cycles of transitions, for example, 30 years in the example demonstrated in Table 1. These calculations can be easily and quickly conducted using spreadsheet software such as Microsoft Excel. This example, although unrealistic because it ignores death, tells us that over half (546 of 1000 = 54.6%) of patients with hepatitis C cirrhosis will have developed HCC after 30 years of follow-up.

The next example shown in Fig. 5 is a slight modification of the first model in that it includes death. In this model, death can occur in two different ways, as indicated by the two arrows leading to the death state in the figure. They include deaths from complications of cirrhosis and those from HCC. In the Degos paper, the annualized probability of death among patients with HCC was 60%, and that among those with cirrhosis but no HCC was 3% [4].

In Table 2, at time zero, the cohort starts 1000 individuals, all with compensated cirrhosis. After the first year, 26 develop HCC (same as the preceding example) and 30 deaths will have occurred from non-HCC cause (1000 × 3%). Things become a bit complicated in the second year, because deaths can occur not only among the 944 non-HCC cirrhotics, but also among the 26 with HCC. Thus, during the second year, 28 non-HCC patients die (944 × 3%), whereas an additional 16 patients (26 × 60%) will die from HCC. Together, 44 deaths will occur during the second year, leading to a total of 74 deceased in the first and second years combined. Meanwhile, 25 (944 × 2.6%) patients

Table 2
A simple three-stage Markov model describing transitions among cirrhosis, HCC, and death

| Year | Cirrhosis | HCC | Death |
|---|---|---|---|
| Zero | 1000 | 0 | 0 |
| 1 | 944 | 26 | 30 |
| 2 | 891 | 35 | 74 |
| — | — | — | — |
| 10 | 562 | 27 | 411 |
| 20 | 316 | 15 | 669 |
| 30 | 178 | 8 | 814 |

Table 3
Comparison of two strategies between no screening and screening for HCC

| | Original model | | | Model with reduced mortality from HCC | | |
|---|---|---|---|---|---|---|
| Year | Cirrhosis | HCC | Death | Cirrhosis | HCC | Death |
| Zero | 1000 | 0 | 0 | 1000 | 0 | 0 |
| 1 | 944 | 26 | 30 | 944 | 26 | 30 |
| 2 | 891 | 35 | 74 | 891 | 43 | 66 |
| — | — | — | — | — | — | — |
| 10 | 562 | 27 | 411 | 562 | 57 | 381 |
| 20 | 316 | 15 | 669 | 316 | 34 | 651 |
| 30 | 178 | 8 | 814 | 178 | 18 | 804 |

The left panel is the same as Table 2. In the right panel, the transition probability from HCC to death is reduced by 50%, by assuming screening for HCC will detect early HCC allowing effective treatment.

develop new HCC and are added to the surviving group with HCC. This leads to a total of 35 patients with HCC at the end of the second year, including 10 (26 − 16) surviving patients who had developed HCC during the first year and 25 with newly developed HCC. This leaves 891 patients, that is, 944 less 28 deaths and 25 developing HCC, remaining in the cohort with cirrhosis at the end of the second year. Although this process is somewhat complicated to describe verbally, the calculation can be undertaken on a spreadsheet fairly easy, which can then be replicated over the period of analysis.

When this process is continued for 30 years, the composition of the cohort appears markedly different from the previous example in Table 3, which highlights the importance of defining states and transitions correctly.

## Sensitivity analysis

One of the most useful features of decision analytic models is that it allows evaluating hypothetical "what if" scenarios. Let us suppose that there is an intervention that reduces mortality in HCC patients by one half (transition probability from HCC to death decreasing from 60 to 30%). An example of such may be a screening program that will detect HCC at an early stage, thereby allowing effective treatment in a larger number of patients, although whether 50% reduction in mortality can be achieved with screening in real life may be debatable.

Table 3 illustrates how the outcome changes when the mortality rate from HCC is reduced. The left panel is identical to Table 2, and is repeated here for easy comparison with the right panel, which is constructed the same way as the left, except that the probability of death among patients with HCC was reduced to 30%.

Fig. 6 compares the two models over a 30-year period. One notes that the difference between the two models is quite small, indicating that reducing the mortality from HCC by 50% does not have a huge impact on survival of the

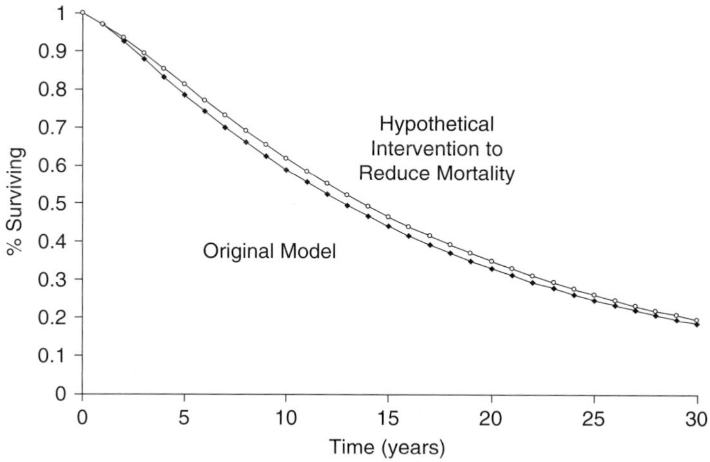


Fig. 6. Comparison of survival curves of the two strategies compared in Table 3.

overall cohort. This may well be the reason why it has been difficult to show the efficacy of screening for HCC. Although HCC is a major threat to patients with cirrhosis, its absolute incidence is still quite low, and it still carries high mortality, with or without screening. One may recall the previous example shown in Fig. 2, which demonstrated a similar point. Thus, to empirically detect the kind of small improvement in survival suggested in Fig. 6, the study will have to be based on a very large number of patients followed over at least a decade.

One may also note that the overall survival appears quite favorable (some patients with cirrhosis surviving longer than 30 years). This is in part due to the fact that the model did not incorporate deaths from causes other than cirrhosis or HCC.

Similar to the consideration of the impact of a hypothetical treatment, one can also vary the value of other input variables in decision analytic models. For example, what would the impact of the treatment be, if the incidence of HCC increases from the current 2.6% per annum to 5%? What if the mortality of cirrhosis decreased from 3% to 1% per year? These questions may be answered almost instantaneously, as most Markov models are created using a computer. Sensitivity analysis is a very useful feature of decision analytic models, as it provides information about the "robustness" of the conclusions reached by the model [1].

## Published examples for decision analytic models in HCC

There have been a number of analyses evaluating the outcome of HCC using decision analytic methods. Some of these addressed screening for HCC in high-

Table 4
Comparison of three decision analyses addressing the effectiveness of screening for HCC

| | Arguedas [5] | Saab [6] | Lin [7] |
|---|---|---|---|
| Model | Markov | Markov | Markov |
| Target population for screening | 50 year olds with cirrhosis (20% decompensated) | LT candidates (decompensated cirrhosis) | 40 year olds with compensated hepatitis C cirrhosis |
| Incidence of HCC[a] | 1.4% (compensated)<br>4% (decompensated) | 2% | 2% (beginning of follow-up)<br>10% (after 8 years of follow-up) |
| Mortality from decompensated cirrhosis[a] | 30% | 3% (UNOS status 3)<br>14% (UNOS status 2A) | 21% |
| Mortality from untreatable HCC[a] | 90% | 90% | 96% |
| Treatment modality | Resection or OLT<br>Loco-regional Tx | OLT<br>Loco-regional Tx | Resection<br>Loco-regional Tx |
| Screening modality | No screening<br>AFP alone<br>AFP + US[b]<br>AFP + CT[b]<br>AFP + MRI[b] | AFP alone<br>US alone<br>AFP + US<br>CT alone | No screening<br>AFP + US q 6mo<br>AFP + US q 12mo<br>AFP q 6mo + US q 12 mo |
| Preferred strategy | AFP + CT | US alone | AFP+US q 6 mo |
| Average increase in life expectancy by preferred strategy | 0.31 (compared to no screening) | 0.007 (compared to AFP alone) | 0.42 (compared to no screening) |

[a] Annual transition probabilities.
[b] AFP and imaging alternated every 6 months.

risk populations, while others tried to identify optimal strategies, for example, liver transplantation for patients diagnosed with HCC. Table 4 compares three recently published models that evaluated screening for HCC [5–7].

First, one may note that although the same modeling technique (ie, Markov) was used for all three analyses, there are important differences in the selection of target population, treatment modalities considered and screening strategies compared. In addition, many of the numerical data used in models were different in each analysis, which makes direct comparison of their conclusions difficult. As a result of the heterogeneity of the models, the conclusions reached by each analysis differed from one another. Not surprisingly, sensitivity analyses showed that their conclusions were subject to variables such as diagnostic accuracy (sensitivity and specificity) and costs of the screening tests employed. One common theme is that in all three analyses, the gain in life expectancy by screening appears quite small, consistent with the hypothetical examples considered in this review. The model by Saab et al [6] did not consider a no-screening strategy, and thus did not have as much survival gain as the others.

With that caveat, there seems to be a consensus among the analyses is that there is a modest gain in survival when screening for HCC is instituted.

## Limitations of decision analytic models

There are limitations to these analytical methods that must be considered in interpreting results. First, the conclusions of decision analytic models depend on (1) structure of the model and (2) data input. In this context, because our knowledge of the natural history and treatment outcome is less than perfect, inclusion of some assumptions in the model is inevitable. Thus, to the extent that the model's structure and data input are based on the best available evidence, the robustness and usefulness of an analysis are determined by the assumptions embedded in them. Although some assumptions may be entirely defensible, others may not be derived from as firm a source. In that sense, rigorous sensitivity analyses are critically important to investigate the influence of each assumption on the conclusions of the analysis. In some cases, these sensitivity analyses may be considered even more important than the base case itself. As discussed before, sensitivity analyses help determine whether the model is "robust" to variations in the assumptions, or whether clinically reasonable changes in assumptions result in different conclusions. If sensitivity analyses reveal that there is a large degree of uncertainty about a key assumption, it points to the need to conduct better designed studies, to obtain more precise data.

One important, yet often ignored, assumption that underlies Markov models is known as the Markovian assumption [8]. This is stated that knowing only the present state of health of a patient is sufficient to project the entire trajectory of future states. In other words, all patients in a given state at a given time are considered to have the same prognosis, no matter how they reached the present state. In the previous example (Table 2), at the end of the second year, there were 35 patients with HCC. These include 25 new patients (those who develop HCC during the second year) as well as 10 existing patients (HCC developed in the first year, but continuing to survive). Subsequent survival in these two groups of patients is likely different from one another. As time progresses, the HCC group becomes quite heterogeneous with respect to the duration of harboring HCC lesions, which may affect individual's probability of death in the ensuing year. Our model completely ignored this fact and applied an identical probability of death in all patients with HCC. This "absence of memory" built into the model almost always represents some degree of departure from reality, although the extent to which that affects the conclusion of the model may not necessarily be significant. It may be possible to construct models to do away with this assumption explicitly, although they tend to result in models that are extremely complex and require additional assumptions.

Finally, some models, as shown in this review, may represent oversimplification of complex medical events that occur in real life. One of the challenges to the analyst is to construct the model in a manner that incorporates all the factors relevant to the clinical question and yet at the same time avoid unnecessary complexities that are immaterial to the conclusion. In fact, inclusion of many minor variables, especially when not based on firm clinical data, may simply lead to unreliable results. For this reason, complete disclosure of the structure of a model and assumptions is essential for validation of its conclusions.

## Summary

Decision analysis helps evaluate competing strategies under conditions of uncertainty in a wide variety of clinical settings. Despite some limitations, decision trees and Markov models remain essential tools for medical decision analysts. These techniques allow comparison of competing management strategies in a quantitative fashion. Sensitivity analysis is an important feature of decision analytic models that identify important factors that affect the outcome of decisions under considerations. Judiciously used, decision analytic models allow a quantitative evaluation of existing data as they relate to strategies ranging from optimizing clinical management at the patient level to allocating health care resources at the societal level.

## References

[1] Pauker SG, Kassirer JP. Decision analysis. N Engl J Med 1987;316(5):250–7.
[2] Petitti D. Meta-analysis, decision analysis and cost-effectiveness analysis. New York: Oxford University Press; 1994.
[3] Beck JR, Pauker SG. The Markov process in medical prognosis. Med Decis Making 1983; 3(4):419–58.
[4] Degos F, Christidis C, Ganne-Carrie N, et al. Hepatitis virus related cirrhosis: time to occurrence of hepatocellular carcinoma and death. Gut 2000;47(1):131–6.
[5] Arguedas MR, Chen VK, Eloubeidi MA, et al. Screening for hepatocellular carcinoma in patients with hepatitis C cirrhosis: a cost–utility analysis. Am J Gastroenterol 2003;98:679–90.
[6] Saab S, Ly D, Nieto J, et al. Hepatocellular carcinoma screening in patients waiting for liver transplantation: a decision analytic model. Liver Transplant 2003;9:672–81.
[7] Lin OS, Keeffe EB, Sanders GD, et al. Cost-effectiveness of screening for hepatocellular carcinoma in patients with cirrhosis due to chronic hepatitis C. Aliment Pharmacol Ther 2004; 19:1159–72.
[8] Sonnenberg FA, Beck JR. Markov models in medical decision making. Med Decis Making 1993;13(4):322–38.

ELSEVIER
SAUNDERS

Clin Liver Dis 9 (2005) 235–251

CLINICS IN
LIVER DISEASE

# Screening Tests for Hepatocellular Carcinoma

Jorge A. Marrero, MD, MS

*Division of Gastroenterology, University of Michigan, 3912 Taubman Center, Ann Arbor, MI 48109-0362, USA*

The decision to screen an at-risk population for cancer is based on well-established criteria [1]. Although the overall goal is to reduce morbidity and mortality from cancer, the objective of screening is the use of a relatively simple, inexpensive test in a large number of individuals to determine whether they are likely or unlikely to have the cancer for which they are being screened [2]. Screening is the one-time application of a test that allows detection of a disease at a stage where curative intervention may improve the goal of reducing morbidity and mortality. Surveillance is the continuous monitoring of disease occurrence (using the screening test) within a population to achieve the same goals of screening [3]. This article will review the process of screening/surveillance for hepatocellular carcinoma (HCC), followed by a discussion on the available screening tests for this tumor.

Criteria have been developed, first promoted by the World Health Organization, to assure the benefits of screening for a specific disease [4]: (1) the disease in question should be an important health problem; its significance may be defined by disease burden, including morbidity and mortality. (2) There should be an identifiable target population. (3) Treatment of occult disease (ie, disease diagnosed before the symptoms appear) should offer advantages compared with the treatment of symptomatic disease. (4) A screening test should be affordable and provide benefits justifying its cost. (5) The test must be acceptable to the target population and to health care professionals. (6) There must be standardized recall procedures. (7) Screening tests must achieve an acceptable level of accuracy in the population undergoing screening. Accuracy

This work was supported by CA864000 Great Lakes New England Clinical Epidemiology Center of the Early Detection Research Network, and DK64909.

*E-mail address:* jmarrero@umich.edu

1089-3261/05/$ – see front matter 
doi:10.1016/j.cld.2004.12.006

***liver.theclinics.com***

will vary by test, cancer site, and individual patient characteristics. We will evaluate the rationale for screening or surveillance of patients with HCC based on these criteria.

## The disease in question should be an important health problem; its significance may be defined by disease burden, including morbidity and mortality

HCC is the fifth most common tumor world wide, with an incidence equal to the death rate [5]. The incidence of HCC has been rising in Europe and the United States [6,7]. A molecular clock study indicated that the epidemic of hepatitis C (HCV) in the United States started in the 1960s and peaked in the late 1980s [8]. Because of the lag time between the onset of infection to the development of cirrhosis, the authors postulate that the incidence of HCV-related HCC will continue to increase over the next 20 years. In addition, the improvement in the survival of patients with cirrhosis due to improved specialty care may further increase the number of individuals at risk for developing HCC.

## There should be an identifiable target population

It has been recognized that the most important risk factor for the development of HCC is cirrhosis, especially in the West [3]. HCV and hepatitis B (HBV) are the major etiologic agents that lead to the development of HCC [9,10]. However, it has been estimated that about 30% of carriers of the HBV surface antigen that go on to develop HCC do not have cirrhosis [11]. HCV is the causative agent that has been responsible for the increase in incidence of HCC in the United States through the development of cirrhosis. Alcoholic cirrhosis is another major etiologic agent leading to HCC. Recently, an association between nonalcoholic liver disease and HCC has been made [12], but there are no cohort studies evaluating the natural history of nonalcoholic fatty liver disease. Other etiologies of chronic liver disease such as hemochromatosis, primary biliary cirrhosis, autoimmune hepatitis, and $\alpha$-1 antitrypsin deficiency are less common causes, with prevalence in HCC between 1% to 8% [13–17].

Other important risk factors for the development of HCC in patients with cirrhosis include male gender, older age, alcohol and tobacco consumption, obesity, and diabetes [18–21]. One study prospectively evaluated factors that independently increased the risk of HCC [22]. They found that prothrombin time $> 75\%$ of baseline, age $> 55$, platelet count $< 75$ mm$^3$, and HCV were independent risk factors for HCC. They stratified patients into a high-risk group (presence of these factors) and into a low-risk group (absence of risk factors), and the 5-year cumulative incidence of HCC was 30% for the high-risk group and 4% for the low-risk group (*P* 0.0001). Further studies should be performed to determine if stratification according to risk is beneficial to target surveillance to high-risk patients.

### Treatment of occult disease should offer advantages compared with the treatment of symptomatic disease

The effectiveness of the treatments for HCC will depend on the stage at the time of diagnosis. Surgical resection has provided 5-year survival rates of 70% in carefully selected patients with preserved hepatic function, no evidence of portal hypertension, and single small asymptomatic tumors (<5 cm in maximal diameter) [23]. However, in Western countries, only about 5% of patients with HCC will be eligible for resection. Liver transplantation is the preferred method of treatment when available, and the HCC is restricted to the Milan criteria, a single nodule <5 cm or <3 nodules each <3 cm in diameter [24]. The 5-year survival reported for liver transplantation is 74% [23]. Ablative treatments (ethanol injection and radiofrequency ablation are the most common modalities used) have 5-year survival rates of 37% when lesions <5 cm are treated [23]. However, the 3-year recurrence rates may exceed 50%, which is similar to surgical resection, and limits the overall efficacy of these treatments. In those with more advanced tumors but preserved hepatic function (intermediate stages) [25], chemoembolization offers 3-year survival rate of 63% in a recent randomized controlled trial [26]. Even though these treatments have shown to improved survival rates, the majority of the studies suffer from lead-time bias. Lead-time bias is the period between early detection of disease and the time of its usual clinical presentation, which merely increases the awareness of their disease without reducing their mortality or morbidity [27]. Mortality rates are not influenced by the timing of diagnosis, whereas median survival or 5-year survival are sensitive to the elapsed time from diagnosis until death, and may be skewed by a screening program. Lead-time bias is an important issue that should be taken into account when determining whether a surveillance program for HCC leads to therapies that improve survival.

### A screening test should be affordable and provide benefits justifying its cost

The standard threshold for cost effectiveness has been determined to be a maximal of $50,000 per quality-adjusted life year (QALY) [28]. Economic models studying the benefits of surveillance programs in HCC have been performed. Surveillance with biannual $\alpha$-fetoprotein (AFP) and ultrasonography in Child class A cirrhotics increase the mean life expectancy with cost-effectiveness ratios between $26,000 and $55,000 per QALY [29]. When a similar analysis was performed in HCV cirrhotics, the cost–utility ratio was $26,689 per QALY [30]. Another study evaluating the cost effectiveness of biannual ultrasound in HCV Child class A cirrhosis showed a cost-effective ratio of $33,083 per QALY [31]. Therefore, screening with ultrasound and AFP has been shown to be cost effective in compensated cirrhotics.

## The test must be acceptable to the target population and to health care professionals

Surveillance of HCC seems to be acceptable to patients with cirrhosis. Such data comes indirectly from cohort studies that have shown that only about 3% to 18% of cirrhotic patients were noncompliant with surveillance using ultrasound and AFP [3], and compares favorably with the 67% noncompliance rate seen with using colonoscopy for colon cancer screening [4]. HCC surveillance also seems to be well accepted by physicians. In a national survey of 554 members of the American Association for the Study of Liver Disease, 84% indicated that they routinely screened patients with cirrhosis for HCC using AFP and ultrasound [32].

## There must be standardized recall procedures

A recent consensus conference offered guidelines on how to investigate abnormalities of the commonly used screening tests (AFP and ultrasound) [33]. If the ultrasound shows a nodule $< 1$ cm in maximal diameter then repeat ultrasound is recommended because the probability of being HCC is low. When the lesion is $\geq 1$ cm, then biopsy of the nodule is recommended because imaging techniques (CT or magnetic resonance imaging) do not have sufficient accuracy to distinguish HCC from other lesions. For nodules $\geq 2$ cm in diameter, imaging tests are more accurate in determining whether a nodule is an HCC. A negative biopsy in these patients does not rule out HCC. An AFP $> 20$ ng/mL was determined to be the cutoff that triggers further testing. Although recall procedures exists, these are not standardized because of the varying expertise in the interpretation and technology of imaging tests throughout medical centers.

## Screening tests must achieve an acceptable level of accuracy in the population undergoing screening

The emphasis on classifying people on the basis of their likelihood of having cancer is the point of cancer screening, because screening tests are not diagnostic tests. Instead, screening tests should distinguish those individuals who may have the disease from the larger group of individuals who most likely do not have it but are at risk for it. The ideal marker for HCC would be specific for HCC and not be detected in premalignant liver disease (ie, cirrhosis regardless of the etiology). It should be easily measurable, and the test should be reproducible, minimally invasive, and acceptable to patients and physicians [34].

Table 1
Phases of biomarker validation in cancer surveillance

| Phases | Type of study | Aims |
|---|---|---|
| 1 | Preclinical exploratory | Promising markers identified |
| 2 | Clinical assay and validation | Assay detects established disease |
| 3 | Retrospective longitudinal | Biomarker detects preclinical disease |
| 4 | Prospective screening | Confirm ability of marker to detect early stage disease |
| 5 | Cancer control | Impact of screening on reducing tumor burden in at-risk population |

Recent developments of gene-expression microarrays, proteomics, and tumor immunology permit thousands of genes and proteins to be screened simultaneously. To establish a formal framework to guide the process of biomarker evaluation and development, a five-phase program is used by the Early Detection Research Network of the National Cancer Institute (Table 1) [35]. Biomarkers are defined as indicators of cellular, biochemical, molecular, or genetic alterations by which normal or abnormal biologic processes can be recognized. Biomarkers include genes, proteins, antibodies, or radiologic tests, and will be the term used to discuss the existing data on screening tests according to these phases.

### *Phase 1: Preclinical exploratory studies*

The aim of phase 1 studies is to identify biologic characteristics unique to HCC that may lead to assays for future clinical use. Studies in this phase are exploratory in nature, using tissue, serum, plasma, or urine, to discover biomarkers that can differentiate HCC from controls. In addition, imaging studies may be used. Finding an expression pattern (high or low) that differentiates HCC from controls is the aim of this phase. If the assay involves continuous variables, then a receiver operating characteristic (ROC) curve should be used, and an optimal cutoff value that will differentiate cases from controls determined [36]. Criteria for the selection of a biomarker for further development have not been established, although it has been suggested that the area under the ROC curve be used for ranking biomarkers.

Table 2 shows a list of potential biomarkers identified at this stage, indicating that these can differentiate those with HCC from those without [37–54]. The results of some of these appear to be promising, such as Glypican-3, but need confirmation in larger studies involving the next phase of biomarker development. Because this is an exploratory phase, the assay is not expected to be standardized, but for the next phase of development the assay should be reproducible and amenable to high throughput.

### *Phase 2: Clinical assay and validation*

For a biomarker to be used as a test for the surveillance of HCC, it requires the sample to be readily available and be obtained noninvasively. Therefore, samples

Table 2
List of HCC markers identified by phase 1 studies

| Phase I markers | Biological material | Sensitivity | Specificity |
| --- | --- | --- | --- |
| Glypican-3 | Tissue | 72 | 100 |
| | Serum | 53 | |
| Pancreatitis-associated antigen | Serum | 40 | 100 |
| p16 methylation | Serum | 81 | |
| Human hepatocyte growth factor | Serum | 100 | 64 |
| Ctokeratin-19 | Serum | 47 | |
| 90K/MAC-2BP glycoprotein | Serum | 46 | 61 |
| Transforming growth factor-beta 1 | Serum | 69 | 66 |
| Lipoprotein (a) | Serum | 44 | |
| Erythrocyte-binding polyamine | Serum | 43 | 92 |
| Tissue polypeptide specific antigen | Serum | 73 | 71 |
| C-reactive protein | Serum | 48 | 58 |
| p53 antibodies | Serum | 41 | |
| CD24 gene | Tissue | 66 | |
| Telomerase activity | Tissue | 100 | 50 |
| Prothymosin alfa | Tissue | 82 | |
| Microsatellite DNA analysis | Tissue | 100 | 80 |
| HCC-associated gene 1 | Tissue | 89 | |
| Epidermal growth factor receptor | Urine | 62 | |

should be obtained from serum, plasma, or urine, while assays that rely on tissue will not be applicable. The aims of this phase are to estimate the true and false positive rates for the clinical assay, and to assess the ability of the assay to differentiate patients with HCC, in particular those with early HCC, from at-risk subjects. The assay for the biomarker found in phase 1 should be simple; its intra- and interassay variability studied and ready for high throughput. It is important at this phase to correlate the results of the biomarker with covariates such as demographics, etiology of liver disease, risk factors for HCC, and tumor staging. The design of these studies should be case-controlled studies. The inclusion of an adequate number of cases in the early stage is important to determine the diagnostic capability of the biomarker for early-stage HCC. The controls should be patients in whom surveillance will ultimately be applied, that is, patients with compensated cirrhosis without known HCC. ROC curve should be used to identify an optimal cutoff to determine the true positive and true negative rates. Combination of tests can also be evaluated at this stage. The performance of a new test or assay should be compared with standard tests for screening, AFP in the case of HCC. The sample size at this phase should have sufficient power to allow for random variation of the biomarker assay and for confidence in the results. Several biomarkers have been identified at this stage for HCC.

*α-Fetoprotein*

In 1963, AFP was detected in the blood of mice with transplantable HCC [55], and this was followed by the observation of AFP in the serum of patients with HCC [56]. It is currently the most widely used screening test for HCC. In

Table 3
Cross-sectional studies evaluating various tests for the detection of hepatocellular carcinoma

| Author | Cutoff | No. of HCC cases | Sensitivity | Specificity[a] | Sensitivity | Specificity[a] |
|---|---|---|---|---|---|---|
| AFP[b] | | | | | | |
| Peng | 20 | 205 | 65 | 88 | | |
| Trevisani | 16[e] | 170 | 60 | 90 | | |
| Cedrone | 100[e] | 74 | 25 | 95 | | |
| Soresi | 30[e] | 197 | 65 | 89 | | |
| Lee | 200 | 54 | 53 | 79 | | |
| Nguyen | 20 | 163 | 63 | 79 | | |
| US | | | | | | |
| Okazaki | NA | 24 | 85 | 98 | | |
| DCP[c] | | | | | AFP[f] | |
| Aoyagi | 50 | 245 | 51 | 87 | 61 | |
| Mita | 10 | 91 | 62 | 95 | 47 | 86 |
| Nomura | 40 | 85 | 28 | 96 | 58 | 86 |
| Lamerz | 90 | 154 | 79 | 90 | 58 | 91 |
| Grazi | 50 | 111 | 53 | 88 | 54 | 97 |
| Marrero | 125[e] | 55 | 89 | 95 | 68 | 82 |
| AFP-L3[d] | | | | | AFP[f] | |
| Taketa | 15 | 20 | 75 | 90 | 70 | 100 |
| Khien | 15 | 65 | 96 | 92 | [g] | |
| Yoshida | 10 | 80 | 49 | | 84 | |
| Wang | 35 | 35 | 57 | 89 | [g] | |
| Taketa | 15 | 85 | 53 | 94 | NA | |
| Oka | 15 | 388 | 36 | 93 | 68 | 49 |

*Abbreviations:* AFP, alpha-fetoprotein; AFP-L3, *lens culinaris*-agglutinin reactive fraction of AFP; DCP, des-gamma carboxyprothrombin; NA, not available; US, ultrasound.

[a] Values expressed as %.
[b] all AFP values expressed as ng/mL.
[c] all DCP values expressed as mAU/mL.
[d] Values expressed as % of total AFP.
[e] Cutoffs identified by ROC curves.
[f] Included studies in which AFP was compared against DCP and AFP-L3.
[g] all HCC patients had AFP >20 ng/mL.

cross-sectional studies, the sensitivity ranged from 25% to 65% and the specificity from 79% to 95% (Table 3) [57–63]. However, the sensitivities and the specificities vary according to the cutoff established. If the cutoff is established at 20 ng/mL, then the sensitivity and specificity is 87% and 30%, respectively, but if the cutoff is raised to 100 ng/mL and 400 ng/mL, and the sensitivity and specificity varies from 72% to 56% and 70% to 94%, respectively [64]. Three studies have performed ROC curves to determine that the optimal cutoffs for AFP at 30, 16, and 100 ng/mL [57–59]. Therefore, it is unclear which is the best cutoff of AFP for detecting HCC. Another important aspect is that the expression of AFP is affected by ethnicity [62], etiology of liver disease [58], treatment of the underlying liver disease [64], and tumor staging [64].

*Des-gamma carboxyprothrombin*

Des-gamma carboxyprothrombin (DCP) is an abnormal prothrombin protein that is generated as a result of an acquired defect in the posttranslational carboxylation of the prothrombin precursor in malignant hepatic cells [65]. Table 3 summarizes the cross-sectional studies identified at this stage [66–71]. The sensitivities and specificities ranged from 28% to 89% and 87% to 96%, respectively. Of the three studies from Japan, only one showed an improved sensitivity of DCP over AFP but two had better specificities; whereas two of three studies in Western countries had better sensitivities and specificities compared with AFP. Only one of these studies was performed by using ROC curves to determine the performance characteristics [71], which showed that DCP was more sensitive and specific than AFP or the combination of AFP and DCP. Further study of DCP with attention to patients with early-stage HCC is needed.

*Lens culinaris-agglutinin reactive fraction of α-fetoprotein*

Elevation of AFP level may be seen in patients with cirrhosis or chronic hepatitis, and is not always related to HCC. Several variants of AFP with differences in the sugar chain have been identified. One variant, the fucosylated variant, has a high affinity of the sugar chain to lens culinaris. This variant, the lens culinaris-agglutinin reactive fraction (AFP-L3) of AFP has been shown to be more specific for HCC than total AFP [72]. Table 3 summarizes the cross-sectional studies that compared AFP-L3 in patients with HCC versus those with cirrhosis [73–76]. AFP-L3 had sensitivities and specificities that ranged from 36% to 96% and 89% to 94%, respectively. Three studies compared AFP-L3 to total AFP, one study found that AFP-L3 had a higher sensitivity but the specificity was lower. Two studies included only HCC patients with total AFP > 20 ng/mL, one study did not provide results on total AFP; comparisons between the accuracies of AFP-L3 and total AFP in differentiating patients with HCC from those with cirrhosis could not be made in these studies. None of the studies used ROC curves to determine the performance characteristics of AFP-L3. The existing data on AFP-L3 needs further validation before going to the next phase of biomarker development.

Other markers such as monosialylated AFP [77], plasma nitrate/nitrite [78], and human hepatocyte growth factor [79] appear promising, but have been evaluated in only one or two studies and need further study. The current studies identified at this phase have significant heterogeneity with regard to how the performance characteristics (true positive and false positive rates) were determined for the biomarker, especially the lack of use of ROC curves to determine the optimal cutoff. In addition, the majority included patients with advanced HCC to assess the performance of the biomarkers and, therefore, irrelevant for evaluating the difference between early-stage tumors and those with cirrhosis. The patient eligibility criteria and definition of HCC vary widely in the studies reviewed, which limits the assessment of these markers for surveillance. Studies that evaluate the performance of biomarkers in patients with early-stage HCC compared with cirrhotics without HCC as controls should be performed. None of the markers discussed are ready for the next phase of validation.

*Phase 3: Retrospective longitudinal studies*

Studies in this phase aim to evaluate the capacity of the biomarker(s) to detect preclinical disease. These studies involve the collection of specimens from a cohort of patients with cirrhosis who are prospectively followed to determine if the biomarker can detect HCC cases before clinical diagnosis of the tumor. Samples from patients who subsequently developed HCC are retrospectively tested to determine if levels of the biomarker were elevated before HCC was diagnosed using available clinical tools. Studies in this phase should also identify variables (covariates) such as demographics, exposure to alcohol and tobacco, family history, etiology of liver disease, and prior treatment of underlying liver disease that may affect the ability of the biomarker to detect early HCC. Other aims include the comparison of various biomarkers singly and in combination. The data analysis should include ROC curves at different time intervals (6 or 12 months) before clinical diagnosis of HCC and at the time of HCC diagnosis to evaluate the performance of the biomarker(s) in preclinical disease [80]. No biomarker has been identified that satisfies the goals established at this phase, but the following markers have been assessed in prospective studies.

*α-Fetoprotein*

Table 4 shows the prospective cohort studies that evaluated the performance of AFP [81–85]. The sensitivities and specificities for AFP ranged from 39% to

Table 4
Prospective studies evaluating of tests for the detection of hepatocellular carcinoma

| Author | No. of cirrhotics | F/U (mo) | No. of HCC identified | Sensitivity | Specificity[a] | Sensitivity | Specificity[a] |
|---|---|---|---|---|---|---|---|
| AFP | | | | | | | |
| Pateron | 118 | 36 | 14 | 50 | 86 | | |
| Oka | 260 | 38 | 55 | 39 | 76 | | |
| Bolondi | 313 | 56 | 61 | 41 | 82 | | |
| Tong | 602 | 34 | 31 | 65 | 90 | [b]100 | 98 |
| Chalasani | 285 | 15 | 27 | 63 | 87 | [b]59 | 93 |
| DCP | | | | | | AFP | |
| Izunno | 137 | 40 | 35 | 23 | | 54 | |
| Ikonna | 188 | 36 | 14 | 57 | | 71 | |
| Shimauchi | 78 | 48 | 21 | 43 | | 14 | |
| Pateron | 118 | 36 | 14 | 7 | 94 | 50 | 86 |
| Ishii | 734 | 13 | 29 | 41 | 90 | 40 | 62 |
| AFP-L3 | | | | | | AFP | |
| Shiraki | 190 | 72 | 21 | 61 | 90 | NA | |
| Sato | 361 | 36 | 33 | 55 | 68 | | |
| Wang | 1500 | 12 | 22 | 75 | 53 | | |

*Abbreviations:* AFP, alpha-fetoprotein; AFP-L3, lens culinaris agglutinin-reactive AFP; DCP, des-gamma carboxyprothrombin; NA, not available.

[a] Values expressed as %.

[b] Values shown for ultrasound.

65% and 76% to 90%, respectively. Ultrasonography was included in two studies, one of them indicating superiority over AFP for the detection of HCC. There are significant limitations in the design of this studies that limit the interpretation of the performance of AFP for surveillance of HCC. One is that the assessment of the performance characteristics of AFP was performed with baseline data and not at the time of diagnosis or at a set time point (ie, 6 months) before diagnosis. The study by Tong and colleagues was unique because they combined all the AFP measurements during the follow-up period, and then assessed the performance characteristics by ROC curves [84]. They did show that the mean AFP concentration was increasing over time in cirrhosis, indicating that the performance of AFP closer to the time of diagnosis may be better than at baseline. However, the major limitation of their study was that it only included 29% cirrhotics, and did not combine ultrasound and AFP in the analysis. The other potential limitation of these studies is that the number of patients developing HCC is relatively low and is unclear if there was enough power to analyze the performance of AFP. More studies are needed to assess the performance of AFP to detect preclinical HCC.

*Des-gamma carboxyprothrombin*

The studies shown in Table 4 were designed to prospectively follow a cohort of patients with cirrhosis without HCC to determine the incidence of HCC as with AFP [81,86–89]. The sensitivities for detecting HCC ranged from 23% to 57% compared with 14% to 71% for AFP. In the largest study on DCP, 734 patients with cirrhosis were followed for a mean of 13 months (range 7–17), during which HCC was detected in 29 patients. The sensitivity and specificity of DCP at baseline was 41% and 90%, and 40% and 62% for AFP, respectively. Overall, AFP and DCP had equal sensitivity, but DCP had better specificity. However, as previously discussed, the analysis of the performance of DCP was performed at entry and not before or at the time of clinical diagnosis of HCC. More studies are needed to assess the performance of DCP to detect preclinical HCC.

*Lens culinaris-agglutinin reactive fraction of α-fetoprotein*

The sensitivities ranged from 55% to 75% and specificities from 68% to 90%, as shown in Table 4 [90–92]. However, two studies included only HCC patients with elevated total AFP at baseline making it impossible to compare the accuracy of AFP-L3 with total AFP. As with DCP and AFP, the performance characteristics used were ones at entry, and did not evaluate the performance of the test before diagnosing HCC. More studies are needed to assess the performance of AFP to detect preclinical AFP.

Other markers identified in this phase include insulin growth factor-1 [93] and human hepatocyte growth factor [94], but these markers have been evaluated in only one to two studies each, and the results need to be confirmed in larger studies. The currently available data on AFP, ultrasound, DCP, or AFP-L3 at this phase does not provide us with the information as to whether they can detect preclinical HCC. These studies were not designed to assess the performance characteristics of these tests, but to determine the incidence rate of HCC in a cohort. Another important limitation is that the current studies did not correlate the biomarker performance with the outcome data. Specifically, it will be important to know whether a positive screening test was associated with an improved survival or mortality, and if it increased the detection of surgical HCC. Even though the current guideline is to perform surveillance of cirrhotics with ultrasound and AFP, we do not know the performance of AFP at varying intervals before the development of HCC or at the time of diagnosis as has been shown in prostate cancer [80].

*Phase 4: Prospective screening studies*

Studies in phase 4 aim to determine the operating characteristics of the biomarker-based surveillance in the relevant population by determining the cancer detection rate and the false referral rate. Other aims would be to evaluate the stage of the tumors detected and the proportion of patients with tumors amenable to curative treatment, to assess the feasibility and costs of implementing the surveillance program, and to monitor for tumors that may be missed. Ideally, phase 4 studies involve randomization to surveillance with the new biomarker versus the standard of care. Because the incidence rate of HCC among cirrhotics is relatively low (1–5% per year), a large sample size will be required for this kind of study. No phase 4 study was found in cirrhotics, but a randomized trial was found in HBV carriers.

A randomized control trial was performed in men who were chronic HBV carriers in the county of Qidong, China [95]. A total of 5581 males age 30 to 69 were randomized to screening with AFP every 6 months (n = 3712) and no screening (n = 1869). After a mean follow-up of 61.9 months, 257 HCCs were diagnosed in those screened versus 117 in those not screened. The cutoff for AFP was 20 ng/mL. Stage I HCC was diagnosed in 28% of screened individuals versus 6% of those not screened. The sensitivity and specificity of AFP was 55% and 87%, respectively. Overall survival was not different among the groups because of the lack of effective treatment in this area. This is the first study randomized control study of screening for HCC in an at-risk population.

As new biomarkers with promising results become available and progress to this phase, a phase 4 study that involves randomization of patients with cirrhosis to surveillance with AFP and ultrasound versus a new biomarker would be warranted.

*Phase 5: Cancer control studies*

Studies in phase 5 aim to determine whether surveillance of an at-risk population using the new biomarker reduces the cancer burden compared with no surveillance. The logistics such as large sample size and long duration required, costs of the study, acceptability by patients and physicians, ethical considerations, and adherence to protocol including no surveillance in the control group make phase 5 studies extremely challenging. No phase 5 study has yet been conducted for HCC.

## Summary

HCC meets most of the criteria established for a cancer surveillance program. It is a common health care problem, a target population is identified, effective treatments are available, recall strategies are in place, and surveillance of cirrhotics is cost effective. The main problem with surveillance for HCC is the lack of acceptable accuracy of the current available screening test in the population studied. As reviewed in this article, the current available literature on AFP is fraught with limitations. Most of the studies were not powered to assess the performance of markers as surveillance tests for HCC. The performance of the AFP assay such as reproducibility was seldom described. Analyses of covariates such as demographics and etiology of liver disease were rarely performed. As a consequence, most new biomarkers for HCC have remained stagnant in phase 1 or 2 studies even though some were first reported as potential HCC markers more than 15 years ago. The prospective studies reviewed evaluated AFP at the time of entry into the study and not around the time of HCC development, which is critical to know the performance of the marker in surveillance. Another limitation of the data is the lack of outcomes to eliminate the possibility of lead time bias with screening with AFP. This is likely related to the lack of randomized control trials to compare markers. Two recent independent studies assessed the quality of AFP as a screening test for HCC [96,97]. They all indicate the lack of data regarding the effectiveness of AFP for the surveillance of HCC for many of the reasons outlined above. Although surveillance of cirrhotics with AFP and ultrasound is recommended, shown to be cost effective, and widely performed, the current data regarding the performance of AFP as a surveillance test for HCC are poor.

Several markers, including glypican-3, DCP, AFP-L3, insulin growth factor-1, and human hepatocyte growth factor, appear to be promising, and should be further evaluated in properly designed phase 2 studies to determine their ability to diagnosed early stage HCC, followed by phase 3 studies that will retrospectively determine if they can detect preclinical disease. If the results hold up, phase 4 studies will prospectively assess their ability to detect asymptomatic HCC.

For progress to be made in the validation of current or new markers, several issues need to be addressed. One is identifying the target population for which the surveillance test will be applied. It is unlikely that a single marker will be effective for the surveillance of HCC in all etiologies. Therefore, as the marker(s) progresses through the phases of validation careful attention to the design of the study should be made regarding the eligibility of patients, that is, cirrhotics or HBsAg carriers, viral versus nonviral etiologies, attention to ethnicities, and the focus on early stage HCC. Second, there is an urgent need for a widely accepted prognostic staging system for HCC so there is homogeneity in the studies throughout the world, especially at phases 1 and 2. The five phases used of biomarker development help to evaluate the published literature and to organize biomarker development so that precious specimen resources and funding can be allocated in a rational manner. This structured approach will be important, as many new biomarkers are likely to be discovered based on gene microarray, proteomics, and tumor immunology during the next decade.

## References

[1] Cole P, Morrison AS. Basic issues in population screening for cancer. J Natl Cancer Inst 1980;64:1263–72.
[2] Smith RA. Screening fundamentals. J Natl Cancer Inst Monogr 1997;22:15–9.
[3] Collier J, Sherman M. Screening for hepatocellular carcinoma. Hepatology 1998;27:273–8.
[4] Meissner HI, Smith RA, Rimer BK, et al. Promoting cancer screening: learning from experience. Cancer 2004;101:1107–17.
[5] World Health Organization 2000. World health statistics annual. Geneva: WHO; 2001.
[6] Bosch X, Ribes J, Borras J. Epidemiology of primary liver cancer. Semin Liver Dis 1999; 19:271–85.
[7] El-Serag HB, Davila JA, Petersen NJ, et al. The continuing increase in the incidence of hepatocellular carcinoma in the United States: an update. Ann Intern Med 2003;139(10): 817–23.
[8] Tanaka Y, Hanada K, Mizokami M, et al. A comparison of the molecular clock of hepatitis C virus in the United States and Japan predicts that hepatocellular carcinoma incidence in the United States will increase over the next two decades. Proc Natl Acad Sci USA 2002;99(24):15584–9.
[9] Beasley RP, Hwang LY, Lin CC, et al. Hepatocellular carcinoma and hepatitis B virus: a prospective study of 22,700 men in Taiwan. Lancet 1981;2:1129–33.
[10] Colombo M, Kuo G, Choo Q, et al. Prevalence of antibodies to hepatitis C virus in Italian patients with hepatocellular carcinoma. Lancet 1989;2:1006–8.
[11] Sakuma K, Saitoh N, Kasai M, et al. Relative risk of death due to liver disease among Japanese male adults having various statuses for hepatitis Bs and e antigen/antibody in serum: a prospective study. Hepatology 1988;8:1642–6.
[12] Marrero JA, Fontana RJ, Su GL, et al. NAFLD may be a common underlying liver disease in patients with hepatocellular carcinoma in the United States. Hepatology 2002;36(6):1349–54.
[13] Deugnier Y, Turlin B. Iron and hepatocellular carcinoma. J Gastrohepatol 2001;16:491–4.
[14] Farinati F, Floreani A, De Maria N, et al. Hepatocellular carcinoma in primary biliary cirrhosis. J Hepatol 1994;21(3):315–6.
[15] Nishiyama R, Kanai T, Abe J, et al. Hepatocellular carcinoma associated with autoimmune hepatitis. J Hepatobiliary Pancreat Surg 2004;11(3):215–9.
[16] Propst T, Propst A, Dietze O, et al. Prevalence of hepatocellular carcinoma in alpha-1 antitrypsin deficiency. J Hepatol 1994;21(6):1006–11.
[17] Donato F, Tagger A, Gelatti U, et al. Alcohol and hepatocellular carcinoma: the effect of lifetime intake and hepatitis virus infections in men and women. Am J Epidemiol 2002;155: 323–31.
[18] El-Serag HB. Epidemiology of hepatocellular carcinoma. Clin Liver Dis 2001;5(1):1–16.
[19] Kuper H, Tzonou A, Kaklamani E, et al. Tobacco smoking, alcohol consumption and their interaction in the causation of hepatocellular carcinoma. Int J Cancer 2000;85:498–502.
[20] Calle EE, Rodriguez C, Walker-Thurmond K, et al. Overweight, obesity and mortality from cancer in a prospectively studied cohort of US adults. N Engl J Med 2003;348:1625–38.
[21] El-Serag HB, Tran T, Everhart JE. Diabetes increases the risk of chronic liver disease and hepatocellular carcinoma. Gastroenterology 2004;126(2):460–8.

[22] Velazquez RF, Rodriguez M, Navascues CA, et al. Prospective analysis of risk factors for hepatocellular carcinoma in patients with liver cirrhosis. Hepatology 2003;37:520–7.
[23] Llovet JM, Bruix J. Early diagnosis and treatment of hepatocellular carcinoma. Ball Clin Gastroenterol 2000;14(6):991–1008.
[24] Mazaferro V, Regalia E, Doci R, et al. Liver transplantation for treatment of small hepatocellular carcinomas in patients with cirrhosis. N Engl J Med 1996;334:693–9.
[25] Llovet JM, Bustamante J, Castells A, et al. Natural history of untreated nonsurgical hepatocellular carcinoma: rationale for the design and evaluation of therapeutic trials. Hepatology 1999; 29:62–7.
[26] Llovet JM, Real MI, Montana X, et al. Arterial embolisation or chemoembolisation versus symptomatic treatment in patients with unresectable hepatocellular carcinoma: a randomised controlled trial. Lancet 2002;359(9319):1734–9.
[27] Gates TJ. Screening for cancer: evaluating the evidence. Am Fam Phys 2001;63:513–22.
[28] Drummond MF, O'Brien B, Stoddart GL, et al. Cost-effectiveness analysis. In: Drummond M, Drummond MF, O'Brien B, et al, editors. Methods for the economic evaluation of health care programmes. 2nd edition. New York: Oxford University Press; 1997. p. 96–138.
[29] Sarasin FP, Giostra E, Hadengue A. Cost-effectiveness of screening for detection of small hepatocellular carcinoma in western patients with Child-Pugh class A cirrhosis. Am J Med 1996;101(4):422–34.
[30] Arguedas MR, Chen VK, Eloubeidi MA, et al. Screening for hepatocellular carcinoma in patients with hepatitis C cirrhosis: a cost-utility analysis. Am J Gastroenterol 2003;98(3):679–90.
[31] Lin OS, Keeffe EB, Sanders GD, et al. Cost-effectiveness of screening for hepatocellular carcinoma in patients with cirrhosis due to chronic hepatitis C. Aliment Pharmacol Ther 2004;19(11):1159–72.
[32] Chalasani N, Said A, Ness R, et al. Screening for hepatocellular carcinoma in patients with cirrhosis in the United States: results of a national survey. Am J Gastroenterol 1999;94(8): 2224–9.
[33] Bruix J, Sherman M, Llovet JM, et al. Clinical management of hepatocellular carcinoma. Conclusions of the Barcelona-2000 EASL conference. European Association for the Study of the Liver. J Hepatol 2001;35:421–30.
[34] Srinivas PR, Kramer BS, Srivastava S. Trends in biomarker research for cancer detection. Lancet Oncol 2001;2:698–704.
[35] Pepe MS, Etzioni R, Feng Z, et al. Phases of biomarker development for early detection of cancer. J Natl Cancer Inst 2001;93:1054–61.
[36] Baker SG. The central role of receiver operating characteristic (ROC) curves in evaluating tests for the early detection of cancer. J Natl Cancer Inst 2003;95:511–5.
[37] Capurro M, Wanless IR, Sherman M, et al. Glypican-3: a novel serum and histochemical marker for hepatocellular carcinoma. Gastroenteroloy 2003;125(1):89–97.
[38] Yamagamim H, Moriyama M, Matsumura H, et al. Serum concentrations of human hepatocyte growth factor is a useful indicator for predicting the occurrence of hepatocellular carcinoma in C-viral chronic liver disease. Cancer 2002;95(4):824–34.
[39] Chuang LY, Hung WC, Tang ML, et al. Urinary epidermal growth factor receptor-binding growth factors in patients with cancers of the digestive tract. Clin Biochem 1994; 27(6):485–9.
[40] Chang YC, Ho CL, Chen HH, et al. Molecular diagnosis of primary liver cancer by microsatellite DNA analysis in the serum. Br J Cancer 2002;87(12):1449–53.
[41] Wu CG, Habib NA, Mitry RR, et al. Overexpression of hepatic prothymosin alpha, a novel marker for human hepatocellular carcinoma. Br J Cancer 1997;76(9):1199–204.
[42] Ivy HN, Wong YM, Lo D, et al. Detection of aberrant p16 methylation in the plasma and serum of liver cancer patients. Cancer Res 1999;59:71–3.
[43] Nakashio R, Kitamoto M, Tahara H, et al. Significance of telomerase activity in the diagnosis of small differentiated hepatocellular carcinoma. In J Cancer 1997;74(2):141–7.
[44] Tu DG, Wang ST, Chang TT, et al. The value of serum tissue polypeptide specific antigen in the diagnosis of hepatocellular carcinoma. Cancer 1999;85(5):1039–43.

[45] Lin ZY, Wang LY, Yu ML, et al. Role of serum C-reactive protein as a markers of hepatocellular carcinoma in patients with cirrhosis. J Gastroenterol Hepatol 2000;15(4):417–21.
[46] Nishiguchi S, Tamori A, Koh N, et al. Erythrocyte-binding polyamine as tumor growth marker for human hepatocellular carcinoma. Hepatogastroenterology 2002;49(44):504–7.
[47] Song BC, Chung YH, Kim JA, et al. Transforming growth factor beta 1 as a useful serologic marker of small hepatocellular carcinoma. Cancer 2002;94(1):175–80.
[48] Iacovazzi PA, Trisolini A, Barletta D, et al. Serum 90K/MAC-2BP glycoprotein in patients with liver cirrhosis and hepatocellular carcinoma: a comparison with alpha-fetoprotein. Clin Chem Lab Med 2001;39(10):961–5.
[49] Basili S, Andreozzi P, Vieri M, et al. Lipoprotein (a) serum levels in patients with hepatocarcinoma. Clin Chim Acta 1997;262(1–2):53–60.
[50] Charuruks N, Tangkijvanich P, Voravud N, et al. Clinical significance of p53 antigen and anti-p53 antibodies in the sera of hepatocellular carcinoma patients. J Gastroenterol 2001;36(12): 830–6.
[51] Zeng JZ, Wang HY, Chen ZJ, et al. Molecular cloning and characterization of a novel gene which is highly expressed in hepatocellular carcinoma. Oncogene 2002;21(32):4932–43.
[52] Nagai T, Murota M, Nishioka M, et al. Elevation of cytokeratin 19 fragment in serum in patients with hepatoma: its clinical significance. Eur J Gastroenterol Hepatol 2001;13:157–61.
[53] Huang LR, Hsu HC. Cloning and expression of CD24 gene in human hepatocellular carcinoma: a potential early tumor marker gene correlates with p53 mutation and tumor differentiation. Cancer Res 1995;55(20):4717–21.
[54] Montalto G, Iovanna JL, Soresi M, et al. Clinical evaluation of pancreatitis-associated protein as a marker of hepatocellular: comparison with alpha-fetoprotein. Oncology 1998;55(5):421–5.
[55] Abelev GI, Perova SD, Khramkova NI, et al. Production of embryonal alpha-globulin by transplantable mouse hepatomas. Transplantation 1963;1:174–80.
[56] Bergstrand CG, Czar B. Demonstration of new protein fraction in serum from the human fetus. Scand J Clin Lab Invest 1956;8:174–81.
[57] Trevisani F, D'Intino PE, Morselli-Labate AN, et al. Serum alpha fetoprotein for diagnosis of hepatocellular carcinoma in patients with chronic liver disease: influence of HBsAg and anti-HCV status. J Hepatol 2001;34:570–5.
[58] Cedrone A, Covino M, Caturelli E, et al. Utility of alpha-fetoprotein in the screening of patients with virus-related chronic liver disease: does different etiology influence AFP levels in HCC? A study in 350 western patients. Hepatogastroenterology 2000;47(36):1654–8.
[59] Soresi M, Magliarisi C, Campagna P, et al. Usefulness of alpha-fetoprotein in the diagnosis of hepatocellular carcinoma. Anticancer Res 2003;23:1747–53.
[60] Peng YC, Chan CS, Chen GH. The effectiveness of serum alpha-fetoprotein level in anti-HCV positive patients for screening hepatocellular carcinoma. Hepatogastroenterology 1999; 46:3208–11.
[61] Lee HS, Chung YH, Kim CY. Specificities of serum alpha-fetoprotein in HBsAg + and HBsAg- patients in the diagnosis of hepatocellular carcinoma. Hepatology 1991;14(1):68–72.
[62] Nguyen MH, Garcia RT, Simpson PW, et al. Racial differences in effectiveness of alpha-fetoprotein for diagnosis of hepatocellular carcinoma in hepatitis C virus cirrhosis. Hepatology 2002;36(2):410–7.
[63] Okazaki N, Yoshida T, Yoshino M, et al. Screening of patients with chronic liver disease for hepatocellular carcinoma by ultrasonography. Clin Oncol 1984;10(3):241–6.
[64] Johnson PJ. The role of serum alpha-fetoprotein estimation in the diagnosis and management of hepatocellular carcinoma. Clin Liver Dis 2001;5(1):145–59.
[65] Ono M, Ohta H, Ohhira M, et al. Measurement of immunoreactive prothrombin precursor and vitamin-K dependent gamma-carboxylation in human hepatocellular carcinoma tissues: decreased carboxylation of prothrombin precursor as a cause of des-gamma-carboxyprothrombin synthesis. Tumour Biol 1990;11:319–26.
[66] Aoyagi Y, Oguro M, Yanagi M, et al. Clinical significance of simultaneous determination of alpha-fetoprotein and des-gamma carboxyprothrombin in monitoring recurrence in patients with hepatocellular carcinoma. Cancer 1996;77:1781–6.

[67] Mita Aoyagi Y, Yanagi M, Suda T, et al. The usefulness of determining des-gamma carboxyprothrombin by sensitive enzyme immunoassay in the early diagnosis of patients with hepatocellular carcinoma. Cancer 1998;82:1643–8.
[68] Nomura F, Ishijima M, Kuwa K, et al. Serum des-gamma carboxyprothrombin levels determined by a new generation of sensitive immunoassay in patients with small-sized hepatocellular carcinoma. Am J Gastroenterol 1999;94:650–4.
[69] Lamerz R, Runge M, Stieber P, et al. Use of serum PIVKA-II determination for differentiation between benign and malignant liver diseases. Anticancer Res 1999;19:2489–93.
[70] Grazi GL, Mazziotti A, Legnani C, et al. The role of tumor markers in the diagnosis of hepatocellular carcinoma, with special reference to the des-gamma carboxyprothrombin. Liver Transplant Surg 1995;1:249–55.
[71] Marrero JA, Su GL, Wei W, et al. Des-gamma carboxyprothrombin can differentiate hepatocellular carcinoma from non-malignant chronic liver disease in American patients. Hepatology 2003;37:1114–21.
[72] Taketa K, Sekiya C, Namiki M, et al. Lectin-reactive profiles of alpha-fetoprotein characterizing hepatocellular carcinoma and related conditions. Gastroenterology 1990;99:508–18.
[73] Taketa K, Okada S, Win N, et al. Evaluation of tumor markers for the detection of hepatocellular carcinoma in Yangon General Hospital, Myanmar. Acta Med Okayama 2002;56: 317–20.
[74] Khien VV, Mao HV, Chinh TT, et al. Clinical evaluation of lentil-reactive alpha-fetoprotein-L3 in histology-proven hepatocellular carcinoma. Int J Biol Markers 2001;16:105–11.
[75] Yoshida S, Kurokohci K, Arima K, et al. Clinical significance of lens culinaris agglutinin-reactive fraction of serum alpha-fetoprotein in patients with hepatocellular carcinoma. Int J Oncol 2002;20:305–9.
[76] Wang SS, Lu RH, Lee FY, et al. Utility of lentil lectin affinity of alpha-fetoprotein in the diagnosis of hepatocellular carcinoma. J Hepatol 1996;25:166–71.
[77] Poon TCW, Mok TSK, Chan ATC, et al. Quantification and utility of monosialylated alpha-fetoprotein in the diagnosis of hepatocellular carcinoma with nondiagnostic serum total alpha-fetoprotein. Clin Chem 2002;48:1021–7.
[78] Moriyama A, Tabaru A, Unoki H, et al. Plasma nitrite/nitrate concentrations as a tumor marker for hepatocellular carcinoma. Clin Chem Acta 2000;296:181–91.
[79] Yamagami H, Moriyama M, Tanaka N, et al. Detection of serum and intrahepatic human hepatocyte growth factor in patients with type C liver diseases. Intervirology 2001;44:36–42.
[80] Thornquist MD, Omen GS, Goodman GE, et al. Statistical design and monitoring of the carotene and retinol efficacy trial (CARET). Control Clin Trials 1993;14:308–24.
[81] Pateron D, Ganne N, Trinchet JC, et al. Prospective study of screening for hepatocellular carcinoma in Caucasian patients with cirrhosis. J Hepatol 1994;20:65–71.
[82] Oka H, Tamori A, Kuroki T, et al. Prospective study of alpha-fetoprotein in cirrhotic patients monitored for the development of hepatocellular carcinoma. Hepatology 1994;19:61–6.
[83] Bolondi L, Sofia S, Siringo S, et al. Surveillance programme of cirrhotic patients for early diagnosis and treatment of hepatocellular carcinoma: a cost effective analysis. Gut 2001;48: 251–9.
[84] Tong MJ, Blatt LM, Kao VWC. Surveillance for hepatocellular carcinoma in patients with chronic viral hepatitis in the USA. J Gastroenterol Hepatol 2001;16:553–9.
[85] Chalassani N, Horlander JC, Said A, et al. Screening for hepatocellular carcinoma in patients with advanced cirrhosis. Am J Gastroenterol 1999;94:2988–93.
[86] Izzuno K, Fujiyama S, Yamasaki K, et al. Early detection of Hepatocellular carcinoma associated with cirrhosis by combined assay of des-gamma carboxyprothrombin and alpha-fetoprotein: a prospective study. Hepatogastroenterology 1995;42:387–93.
[87] Ikoma J, Kaito M, Ishihara T, et al. Early diagnosis of hepatocellular carcinoma using a sensitive assay for serum des-gamma carboxyprothrombin: a prospective study. Hepatogastroenterology 2002;49:235–8.
[88] Shimauchi Y, Tanaka M, Kuromatsu R, et al. A simultaneous monitoring of lens culinaris agglutinin A-reactive alpha-fetoprotein and des-gamma carboxyprothrombin as an early

diagnosis of hepatocellular carcinoma in the follow-up of cirrhotic patients. Oncol Rep 2000; 7:249–56.

[89] Ishii M, Gama H, Chida N, et al. Simultaneous measurements of serum alpha-fetoprotein and protein induced by vitamin K absence for detecting hepatocellular carcinoma. South Tohoku District Study Group. Am J Gastroenterol 2000;95:1036–40.

[90] Shiraki K, Takase K, Tameda Y, et al. A clinical study of lectin-reactive alpha-fetoprotein as an early indicator of hepatocellular carcinoma in the follow up of cirrhotic patients. Hepatology 1995;22:802–7.

[91] Sato Y, Nakata K, Kato Y, et al. Early recognition of hepatocellular carcinoma based on altered profiles of alpha-fetoprotein. N Engl J Med 1993;328:1802–6.

[92] Wang SS, Lu RH, Lee FY, et al. Utility of lentil lectin affinity of alpha-fetoprotein in the diagnosis of hepatocellular carcinoma. J Hepatol 1996;25:166–71.

[93] Mazzioti G, Sorvillo F, Morisco F, et al. Serum insulin-like growth factor-1 evaluation as a useful tool for predicting the risk of developing hepatocellular carcinoma in patients with hepatitis C virus-related cirrhosis. Cancer 2002;95:2539–45.

[94] Yamagamim H, Moriyama M, Matsumura H, et al. Serum concentrations of human hepatocyte growth factor is a useful indicator for predicting the occurrence of hepatocellular carcinomas in C-viral chronic liver diseases. Cancer 2002;95:824–34.

[95] Chen JG, Parkin DM, Chen QG, et al. Screening for liver cancer: results of a randomized controlled trial in Qidong, China. J Med Screen 2003;10(4):204–9.

[96] Gupta S, Bent S, Kohlwes J. Test characteristics of alpha-fetoprotein for detecting hepatocellular carcinoma in patients with hepatitis C. Ann Intern Med 2003;139:46–50.

[97] Gebo KA, Chander G, Jenckes MW, et al. Screening tests for hepatocellular carcinoma in patients with chronic hepatitis C: a systematic review. Hepatology 2002;36:S84–92.

ELSEVIER
SAUNDERS

Clin Liver Dis 9 (2005) 253–279

CLINICS IN
LIVER DISEASE

# Imaging Diagnosis of Hepatocellular Carcinoma with Differentiation from Other Pathology

Tae Kyoung Kim, MD*, Hyun-Jung Jang, MD, Stephanie R. Wilson, MD

*Department of Medical Imaging, Toronto General Hospital, University of Toronto, 585 University Avenue, Toronto, Ontario M5G 2N2, Canada*

Hepatocellular carcinoma (HCC) is the most common primary liver malignancy. The majority of HCCs develop in cirrhotic livers. The stepwise development of HCC in a cirrhotic liver is now well recognized; a regenerative nodule (RN) might be the first step in hepatocarcinogenesis, subsequently developing into an HCC through a dysplastic nodule (DN) in a multistep fashion [1,2]. The change of histologic types of the nodule is believed to be sequential; however, the distinctions between each step are not always clear even upon histopathology, which suggests a continuous transition [1]. HCC may also arise de novo from a relatively normal liver without a background of RN or DN, especially in non-Asian populations [3]. The early diagnosis of HCC is important because the most effective treatment is surgical resection or local ablation therapy when the tumor is small.

Over the last few decades there has been remarkable progress of imaging techniques for diagnosing HCC. High-resolution ultrasound (US) scan enables us to detect subcentimeter lesions in the liver. Recent fast CT and magnetic resonance (MR) scanners provide multiphasic contrast-enhanced imaging, which has become a routine imaging technique for cirrhotic livers. The role of arterial phase (AP) imaging is extremely important to detect and characterize focal liver

* Corresponding author.
*E-mail address:* taekyoung.kim@uhn.on.ca (T.K. Kim).


doi:10.1016/j.cld.2004.12.010 *liver.theclinics.com*

lesions in a cirrhotic liver. US scan is most commonly used as a screening test for HCC in high-risk patients. Multiphasic contrast-enhanced CT and MR scans are usually performed when there is any focal lesion suspected of HCC on US or there is a strong clinical suspicion of HCC. However, the use of imaging tests is variable, and depends on institutional preference. In our institution, US scan is most commonly used as a routine screening imaging test for high-risk patients and CT or MR scan is performed to characterize any focal lesions detected on

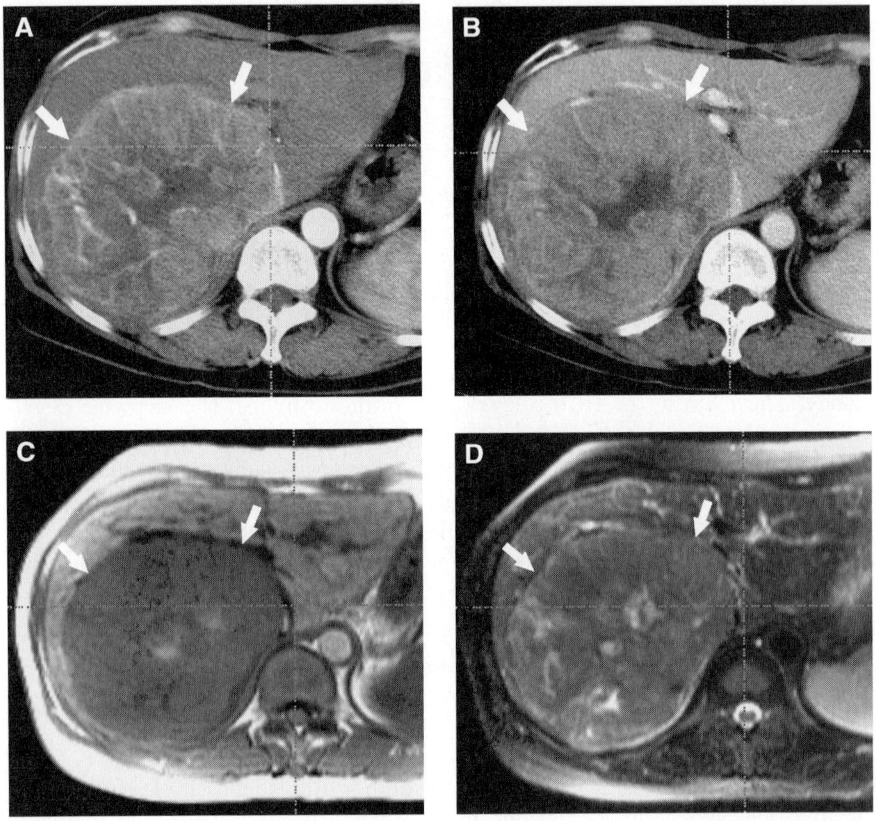


Fig. 1. Expansive HCC. (*A*) An AP CT shows a large, heterogeneously enhancing mass with a well-demarcated margin (*arrows*) in the right hepatic lobe. (*B*) On the portal venous phase CT scan, the mass (*arrows*) shows heterogeneous hypoattenuation with nonenhancing center. The adjacent vessels are stretched by the mass rather than invaded. (*C*) The T1-weighted axial MR image shows hypointense mass (*arrows*) relative to the parenchyma. Note the heterogeneous component in the center with hyperintensity. (*D*) On the axial T2-weighted MR image, the mass (*arrows*) shows heterogeneous hyperintensity with a thin hypointense rim corresponding to a capsule. (*E*) On the delayed phase of the gadolinium-enhanced T1-weighted MR scan, the mass (*arrows*) shows obvious negative enhancement compared with the parenchyma. Note a thin rim enhancement representing a capsule. (*F*) Coronal MR angiography clearly demonstrates a hypervascular mass (*arrows*) with dysmorphic intratumoral arteries. (*G*) Photography of a resected specimen shows a well-encapsulated mass containing areas of necrosis and large intratumoral vessels, well correlated with CT and MR imaging.

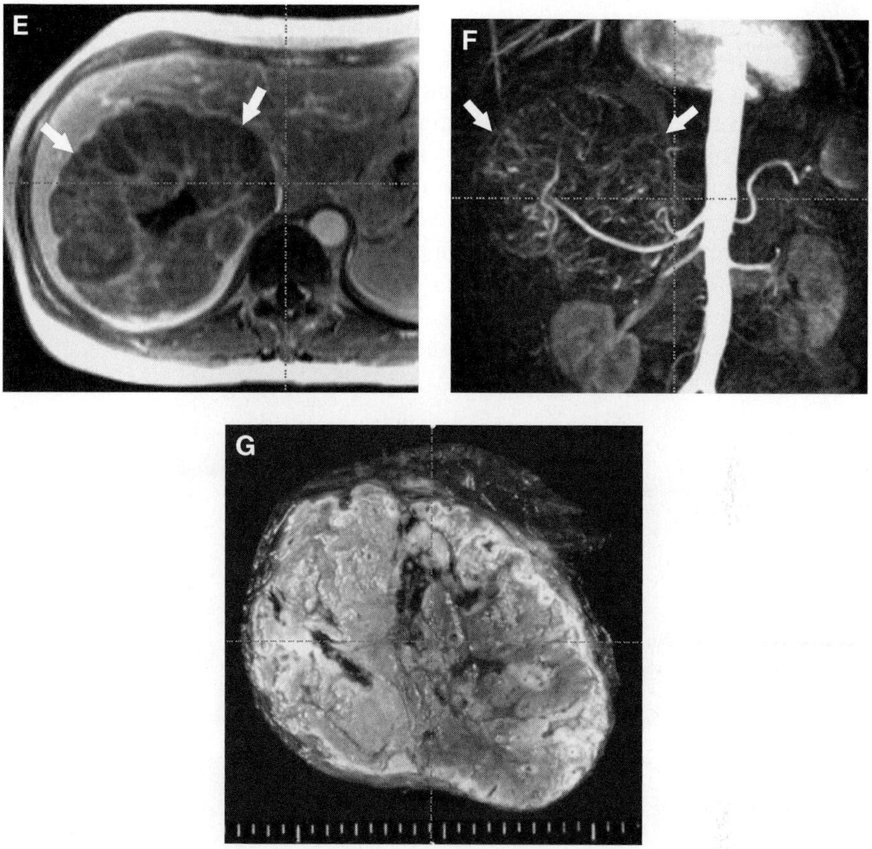


Fig. 1 (*continued*).

US scan. A considerable number of contrast-enhanced US examinations are also performed to characterize small indeterminate focal liver lesions in cirrhotic livers detected on US, CT, or MR scans, producing satisfactory results [4].

Although recent progress of imaging techniques improves the sensitivity to detect HCC, it also reveals a large number of pseudolesions and benign tumors that can mimic the appearance of HCC [5,6]. These lesions can alter the management of the patient, potentially preventing curative surgery. It is, therefore, critical to achieve noninvasive characterization of focal liver lesions with reasonable imaging criteria and adequate additional or follow-up imaging studies. Unfortunately, there are significant overlaps between the imaging findings of benign and malignant liver lesions in cirrhotic livers.

In this article, we review the typical imaging features of HCC and other cirrhosis-related nodules. We also discuss the diagnostic role and accuracy of each imaging test. We focus, in particular, on the difficult imaging diagnosis and characterization of small liver lesions in the cirrhotic liver.

## Typical imaging findings of hepatocellular carcinoma

It is usually easy to make an imaging diagnosis of HCC when the tumor is large if expansive or advanced infiltrative tumors are shown. Expansive HCCs are well-demarcated, nodular, and frequently encapsulated (Fig. 1). On the other hand, infiltrative HCCs have irregular and indistinct margin with frequent invasion of the portal veins or hepatic veins (Fig. 2). A mixed expansive and infiltrative growth pattern is not uncommon (Fig. 3). Expansive HCCs have a

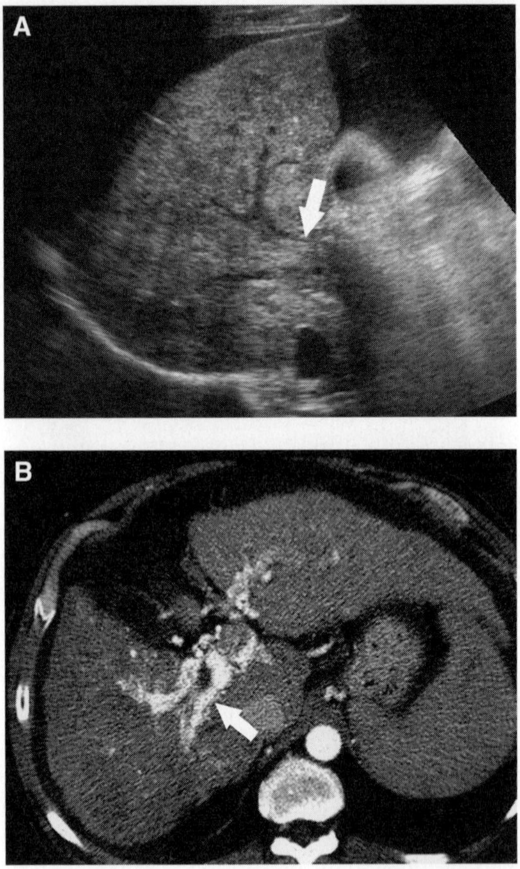


Fig. 2. Infiltrative HCC. (*A*) A sagittal US scan of the right hepatic lobe shows a heterogeneous soft tissue echo replacing and expanding the lumen of the right portal vein (*arrow*). Note a very heterogeneous liver contiguous to the thrombus without definable margin or mass effect. Also noted is a large amount of ascites. (*B*) An AP CT scan shows heterogeneous enhancing thrombus in the portal venous lumen with thick peripheral enhancement as high as that of the aorta (*arrow*). (*C*) An AP CT scan at the level of the main portal vein shows strong enhancement of the main portal vein (*arrow*) as high as that of the aorta, indicating gross arterioportal shunting. (*D*) A portal venous phase CT scan demonstrates ill-defined areas of negative enhancement in the right hepatic lobe and Segment 3, representing infiltrative HCC contiguous to the portal venous thrombi.

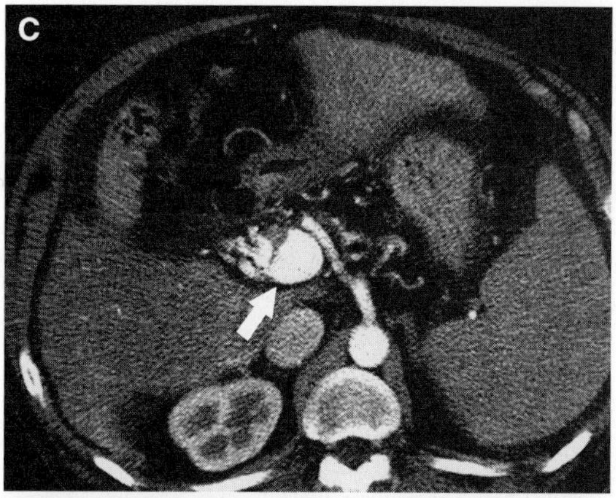


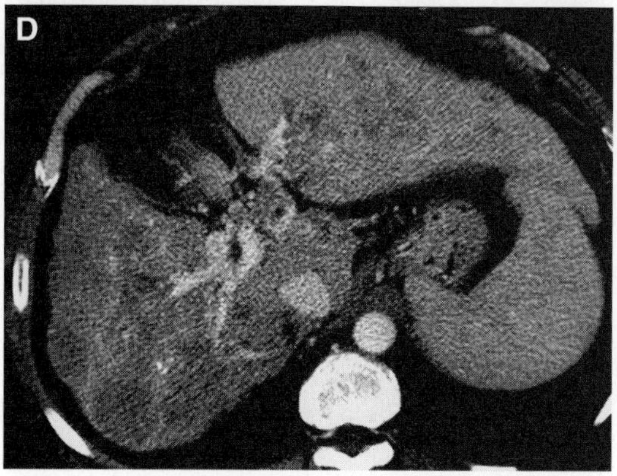


Fig. 2 (*continued*).

better prognosis and better response to the treatment. HCC is distinguished from secondary liver malignancies by its propensity to invade to and grow within the portal vein, hepatic vein, and bile duct. HCC may extend into the inferior vena cava and further into the right atrium (Fig. 4). Extrahepatic metastases of HCC are found anywhere in the body, and mostly occur at an advanced stage, but are infrequently found in small intrahepatic HCC [7]. Intraperitoneal metastasis is an uncommon manifestation of extrahepatic spread, which usually follows rupture of an HCC or prior percutaneous biopsy, local ablation therapy, or surgery (Fig. 4) [8]. With the improvement of imaging techniques and screening programs for HCC, the proportion of small HCCs among the entire group of HCC is increasing as more HCCs are detected in their early stages [9]. However, it is frequently not easy to characterize small focal liver lesions in the cirrhotic liver.

The evaluation of the blood supply in a hepatocellular nodule is extremely important to characterize the lesion because there are sequential changes in the supplying vessels and hemodynamic state during hepatocarcinogenesis. Ad-

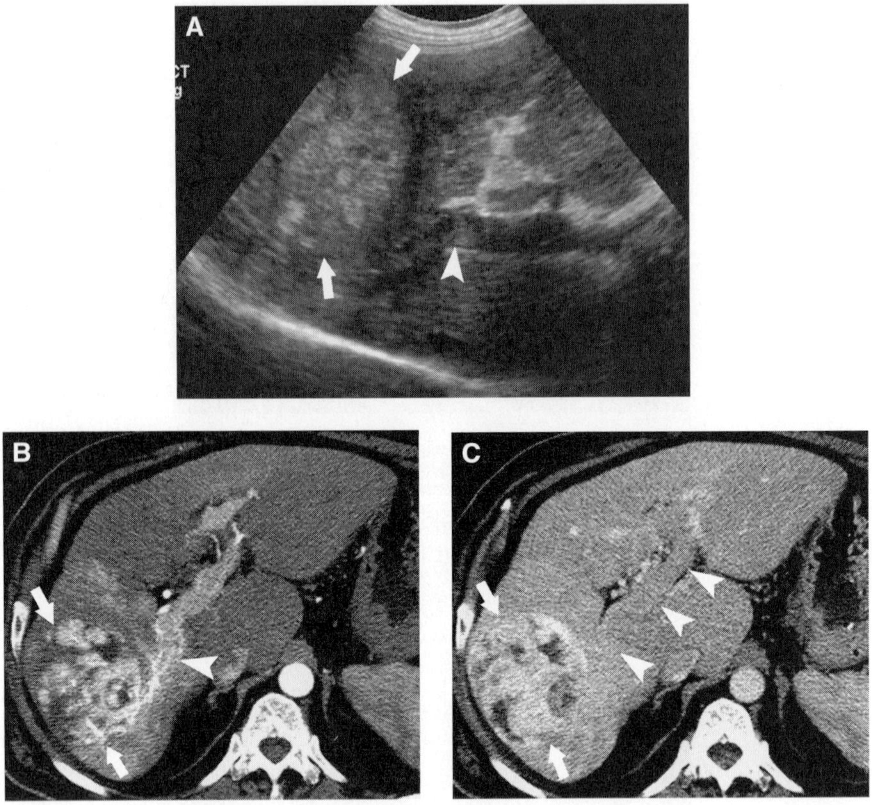


Fig. 3. HCC with mixed expansive and infiltrative growth. (*A*) A transverse US scan shows a heterogeneous mass (*arrows*) with a relatively well-defined anterior margin. Seen is a soft tissue (*arrowhead*) in the right portal vein extending from the mass. (*B*) An AP CT scan shows a heterogeneously enhancing mass (*arrows*) in the right lobe extending into the portal vein all the way to the left portal vein. Note the portal venous thrombi with "thread-and-streak" enhancement (*arrowhead*), which is typical for tumor thrombosis. (*C*) A portal venous phase CT scan shows the portal vein replaced by tumor thrombi (*arrowheads*).

vanced HCCs are typically supplied by abnormal arteries alone (Fig. 5). RNs and DNs usually have normal hepatic arteries and portal veins within the lesion. As DNs have more histologic atypia and malignant changes, abnormal arterial supply increases and normal arterial and portal supply decrease. More specifically, normal portal tracts, including portal vein and hepatic artery, decrease in parallel with an increasing grade of malignancy, and are almost absent in HCCs. In contrast, abnormal arteries due to tumor angiogenesis occur in high-grade DN during the course of hepatocarcinogenesis, and are markedly increased in moderately or poorly differentiated HCCs. Early HCC or well-differentiated HCC have variable degrees of arterial and portal venous supply, making the diagnosis difficult. Moreover, there are significant overlaps of vascular supply between

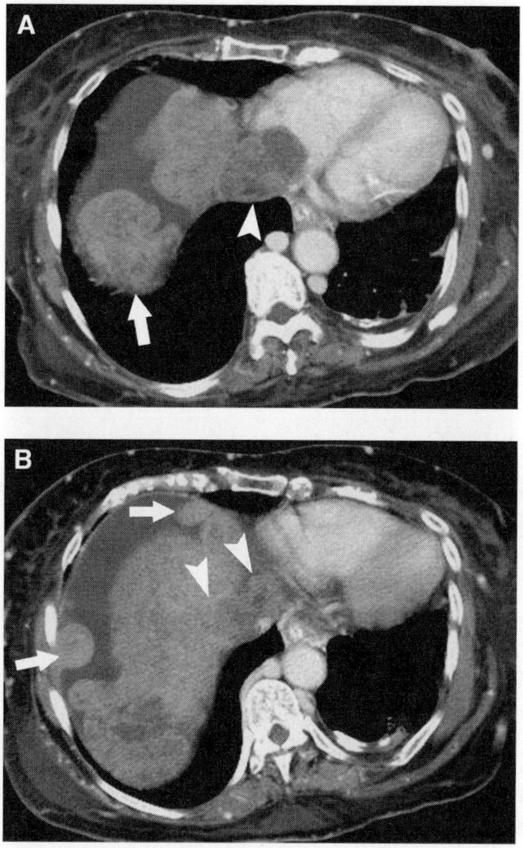


Fig. 4. HCC extending into the inferior vena cava and the right atrium. (*A*) A portal venous phase CT scan shows a heterogeneous attenuating tumor thrombus (*arrowhead*) extending into the right atrium. Noted is a peritoneal mass (*arrow*) with similar appearance to HCC in the liver. (*B*) A portal venous phase CT scan at the level 1 cm caudal to (*A*) shows a tumor thrombus extending into the inferior vena cava (*arrowhead*). Also noted are multiple masses representing peritoneal seeding of HCC (*arrows*).

DNs and well-differentiated HCCs. Some DNs show a decrease in both arterial and portal venous supply, probably due to decreased normal arterial and portal veins without substantial increase of abnormal arteries [10–13].

### *Ultrasound*

HCCs may grow as a solitary or multiple discrete nodules or show as an ill-defined infiltrative mass. Tumors have variable echogenicity on gray-scale US. Small tumors without fatty metamorphosis are usually hypoechoic (Fig. 6), but the echo pattern changes as the size increases. HCC with expansive growth is usually seen as a discrete nodule with a heterogeneous echo, and may have a

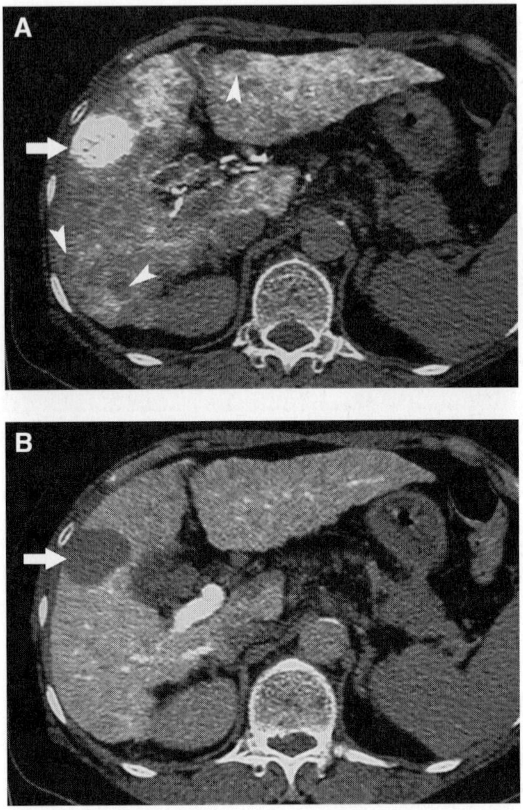


Fig. 5. HCC on angiography-assisted CT scan. (*A*) A CT during hepatic arteriography shows an HCC (*arrow*) with strongly positive enhancement indicating markedly increased arterial flow. Also seen are multiple small nodules (*arrowheads*) with decreased arterial flow likely representing regenerative or DNs. (*B*) On CT during arterial portography, the mass (*arrow*) is seen as a perfusion defect reflecting the lack of a portal venous supply. Note the small nodules noted in (*A*) are not well appreciated, suggesting that those nodules contain similar portal flow compared with the parenchyma.

hypoechoic rim that corresponds to a fibrous capsule (Fig. 7) [14]. In contrast, infiltrative HCC appears as an area with heterogeneous echogenicity, and can be easily overlooked on US scan. It is important to evaluate portal veins within any suspicious heterogeneous area on US because portal vein thrombosis is frequently associated with infiltrative HCC (Fig. 2). Color or power Doppler US is useful to demonstrate the presence of arterial hypervascularity within the mass and the typical morphology of intratumoral and peritumoral vessels, the so-called "basket" pattern [15,16].

A variety of microbubble-based contrast agents are now available for clinical use in many European and Asian countries as well as Canada. But none of these agents has been approved for liver imaging in the United States. Vascularity of

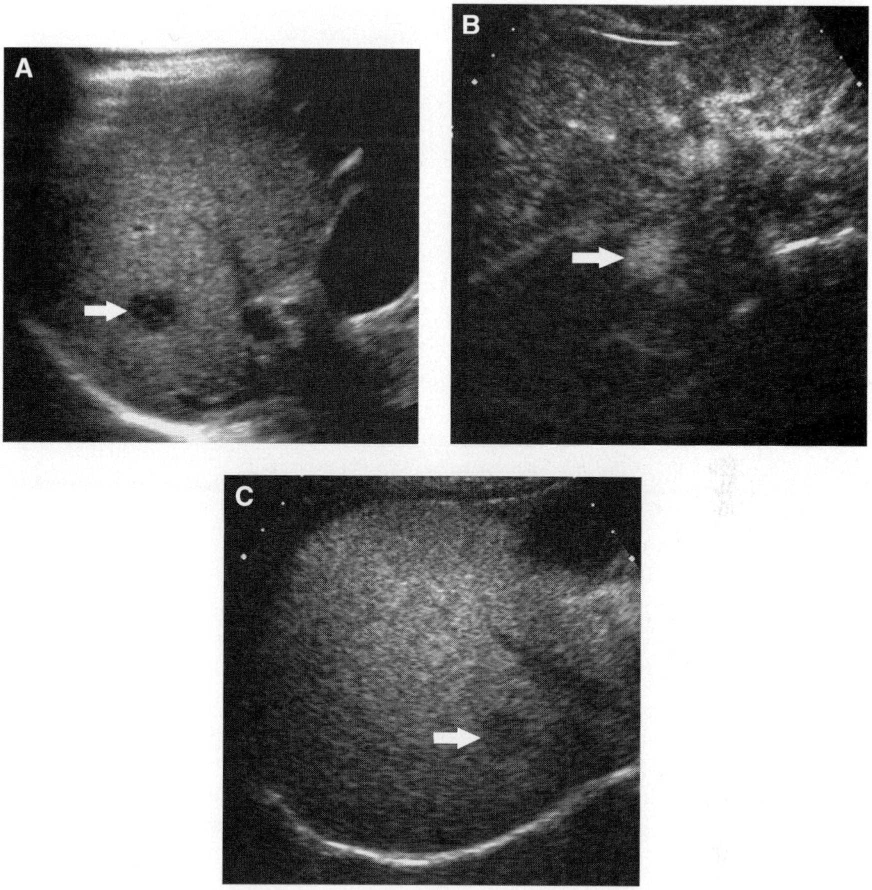


Fig. 6. A small HCC on unenhanced and contrast-enhanced US scan. (*A*) A sagittal US scan shows a 1.5-cm hypoechoic nodule (*arrow*) in the right hepatic lobe. (*B,C*) A contrast-enhanced US scan shows a nodule (*arrow*) with positive enhancement during hepatic AP (*B*) and negative enhancement during the portal venous phase (*C*), which is characteristic of HCC.

HCC can be better evaluated by power Doppler US with a microbubble contrast agent. But the artifactual Doppler signals from contrast agent such as "blooming" artifact or flash artifact are problematic [17]. Use of harmonic power Doppler can decrease these artifactual signals [18,19]. The use of low-mechanical index pulse inversion US imaging with a perfluorocarbon-based contrast agent has markedly improved the diagnostic utility for liver imaging. Our experience shows that contrast-enhanced US is helpful for differential diagnosis of newly detected small liver lesions on screening US or indeterminate lesions seen on CT or MR scans [4,20]. HCCs typically show strong, heterogeneous enhancement with irregular intratumoral vessels on AP scans and negative enhancement

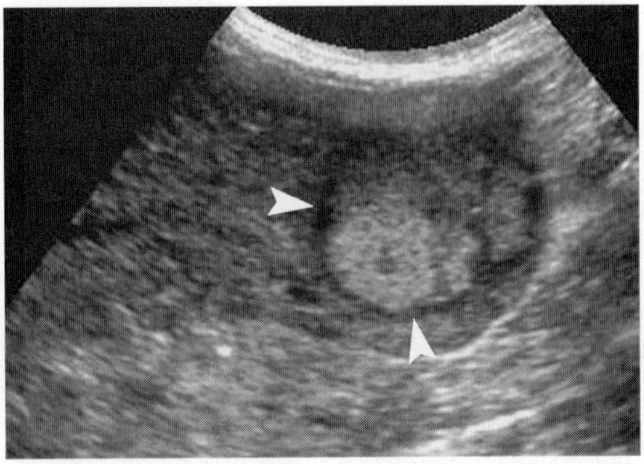

Fig. 7. A typical gray scale US of HCC. A sagittal US scan shows a heterogeneous hyperechoic mass with a hypoechoic rim (*arrowheads*) corresponding to a fibrous capsule.

("washout") compared with the adjacent liver parenchyma on portal or delayed-phase scans (Fig. 8) [4,21–24].

### *CT scan*

The multiphasic CT scan has been established as the standard imaging technique for staging HCC. An AP scan is most important to detect and characterize hypervascular HCCs (Fig. 8) [25–27]. AP scans can also demonstrate hemodynamic changes associated with HCC or liver cirrhosis, such as arterioportal shunting (Fig. 2). It is critical to obtain the optimal AP scan with adequate time delay after the injection of intravenous contrast material [28]. The time delay must be tailored to the type of CT scanner, scanning technique, and the method of administration of contrast material. A portal phase scan is also important to evaluate for venous invasion (Fig. 3), distant metastases, and extrahepatic abnormalities. The attenuation of HCCs on portal phase scan is variable. A delayed-phase scan obtained at least 3 minutes after injection of contrast material is helpful to characterize HCC by demonstrating negative enhancement of HCC compared with the adjacent liver parenchyma (Fig. 9) [29].

### *Magnetic resonance scan*

The signal intensity of HCC on T1-weighted MR scan varies with tumor grade and biochemical composition. Advanced HCCs more frequently show hypointensity than hyperintensity on T1-weighted imaging (Fig. 1). On the other hand, most borderline malignant lesions and the majority of well-differentiated HCCs show hyperintensity. The hyperintensity on T1-weighted images is partly due to fatty metamorphosis in HCCs. The presence of intratumoral fat can be accurately demonstrated by chemical shift MR imaging (Fig. 10). Mild hyperintensity of a nodule in a cirrhotic liver on T2-weighted images is highly suggestive of malignancy (Fig. 10); however, many well-differentiated HCCs are seen as an isointensity or hypointensity [30]. The fibrous capsule is seen as a hypointense rim on both T1- and T2-weighted images. Recent improvements of fast MR imaging techniques allow us to image the entire liver in multiple phases of contrast enhancement. Multiphasic (unenhanced, arterial, portal, and delayed phases) gadolinium-enhanced T1-weighted imaging shows findings similar to those

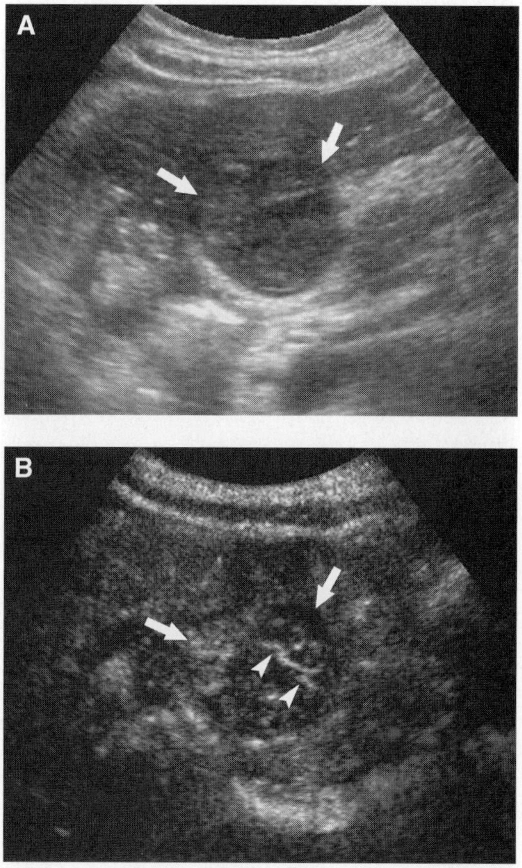


Fig. 8. A typical enhancement pattern of nodular HCC. (*A*) A transverse US scan shows an exophytic mass (*arrows*) with heterogeneous hypoechogenicity. (*B*) An early AP scan of contrast-enhanced US clearly demonstrates dysmorphic intratumoral vessels (*arrowheads*) in the mass (*arrows*). (*C*) On the late AP of the contrast-enhanced US, the mass (*arrows*) shows heterogeneous enhancement. (*D*) On the portal venous phase scan of the contrast-enhanced US, the mass (*arrows*) becomes hypoechoic as the enhancement of the mass washes out. (*E*) An AP CT scan shows heterogeneous positive enhancement of the mass (*arrow*) concordant with contrast-enhanced US (*C*). (*F*) On portal venous phase CT scan, the mass (*arrow*) becomes slightly hypoattenuating to the surrounding parenchyma.

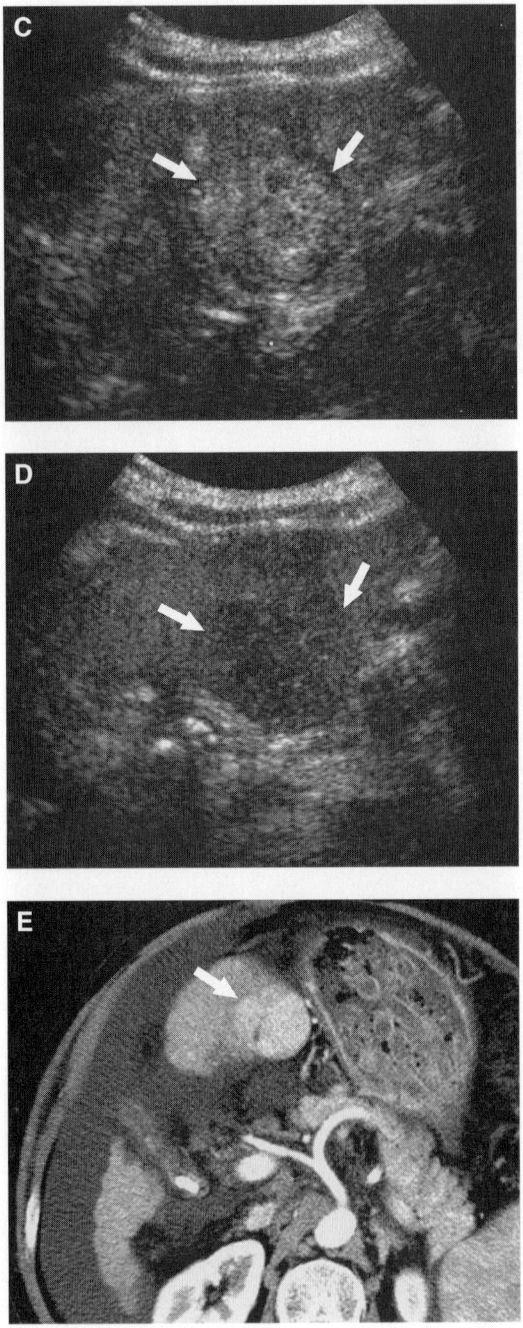


Fig. 8 (*continued*).

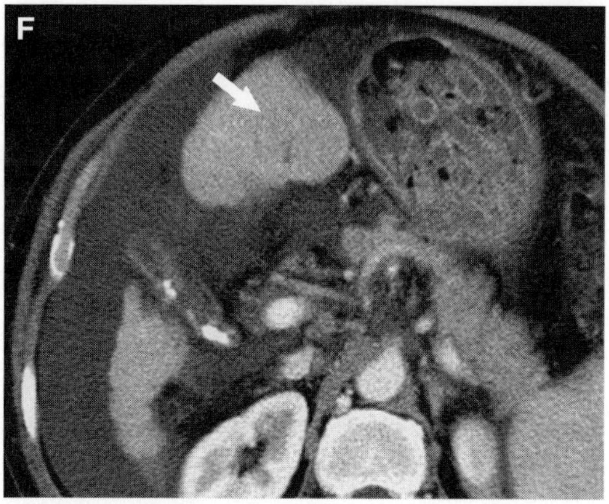


Fig. 8 (*continued*).

of multiphasic contrast-enhanced CT and is most important to detect and characterize HCC in a cirrhotic liver (Fig. 10) [31].

## Dysplastic nodules and regenerative nodules

In a small newly detected nodule in a cirrhotic liver, the differential diagnosis between HCC and other types of cirrhosis-related nodules is important clinically. Percutaneous biopsy under US guidance might be the most accurate diagnostic technique. However, it is occasionally difficult to obtain exact tissue samples from these nodules. Further several difficulties and controversies remain regarding the differential diagnosis of nodules in needle biopsy specimens. Differential diagnosis by imaging findings is therefore important.

Changes of blood supply detected by contrast-enhanced imaging in accordance with the progression from benign hepatocellular nodules to HCC can estimate the grade of malignancy of the nodule. This information is useful clinically to determine the management or additional or follow-up imaging tests. At present, it may be reasonable to estimate the grade of malignancy rather than making a definite differential diagnosis among borderline lesions.

Hepatocellular nodules in a cirrhotic liver are classified as RN, DN, or HCC, as proposed by the International Working Party of the World Congress of Gastroenterology in 1994 [32]. DNs are further classified as low- and high-grade DNs. A DN may contain a microscopic area of HCC, and then called a DN with subfocus of HCC. The distinguishable criteria at each step are the size, cellularity, and the presence of atypia upon histopathology. The distinctions between each step are not always clear, which suggests a continuous transition [1]. These hepatocellular nodules become larger in relation to the grade of malignancy of

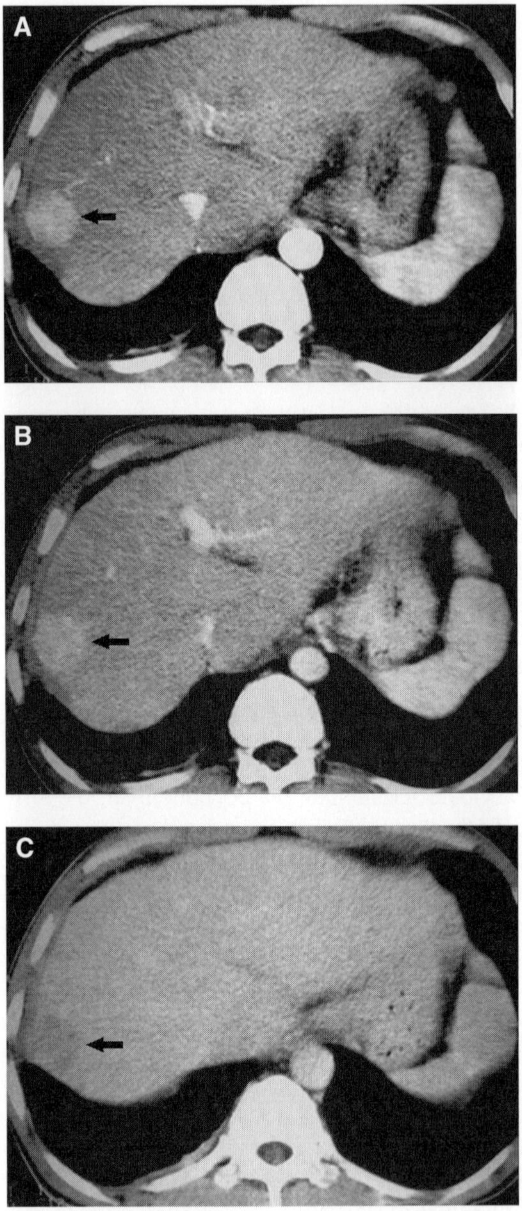


Fig. 9. A delayed washout of contrast enhancement in HCC. (*A*) An AP CT scan shows hypervascular mass (*arrow*) in the periphery of the right lobe. (*B*) During portal venous phase, the mass (*arrow*) shows persistent positive enhancement. (*C*) A CT scan obtained at 3 minutes after the injection of the contrast material clearly demonstrates a heterogeneous washout of contrast enhancement (*arrow*), leading to a confident diagnosis of HCC.

the nodules, although there is a wide range of overlap between the sizes of these different types of nodules.

RNs are small and usually do not stand out on imaging. US scan frequently demonstrates a coarse and heterogeneous echotexture of the liver parenchyma with a nodular surface in cirrhotic livers with RNs. RNs are infrequently seen as numerous tiny hypoechoic lesions throughout the liver on US imaging. CT is not very sensitive to the presence of RNs. Delayed-phase contrast-enhanced CT scan may show RNs as numerous slightly hypoattenuating nodules. Siderotic RNs can be seen as tiny hypointense lesions on gradient-echo MR images due to their iron content (Fig. 11), and may be seen as slightly hyperattenuating lesions on unenhanced CT.

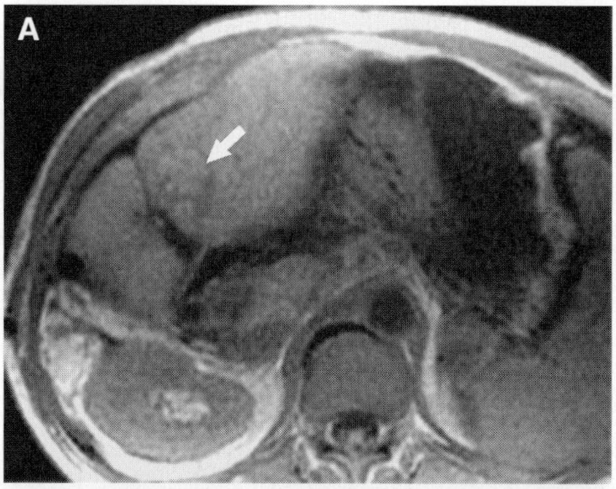


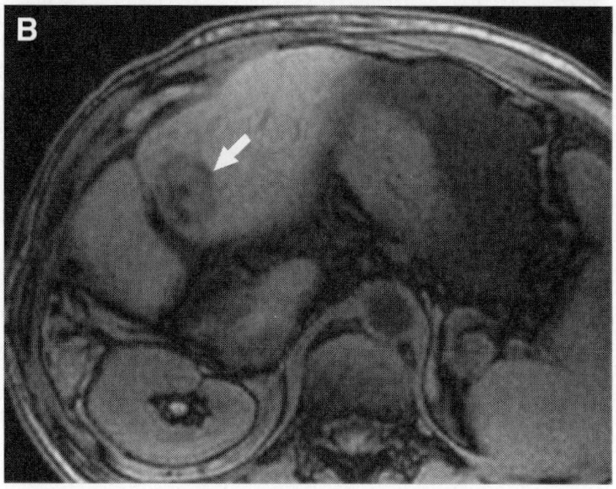


Fig. 10. A fatty metamorphosis of HCC. (*A*) An in-phase T1-weighted MR scan shows a mass (*arrow*) containing areas of slight hyperintensity. (*B*) An out-of-phase T1-weighted MR scan, which reduces the signal from the fat, confirms the presence of intratumoral fat by demonstrating marked reduction of the signal intensity of the mass (*arrow*). (*C–E*) The mass (*arrow*) shows mild hyperintensity on a T2-weighted MR scan (*C*), heterogeneous enhancement on an AP scan (*D*), and a washout on a delayed phase scan (*E*) of dynamic gadolinium-enhanced T1-weighted MR images.

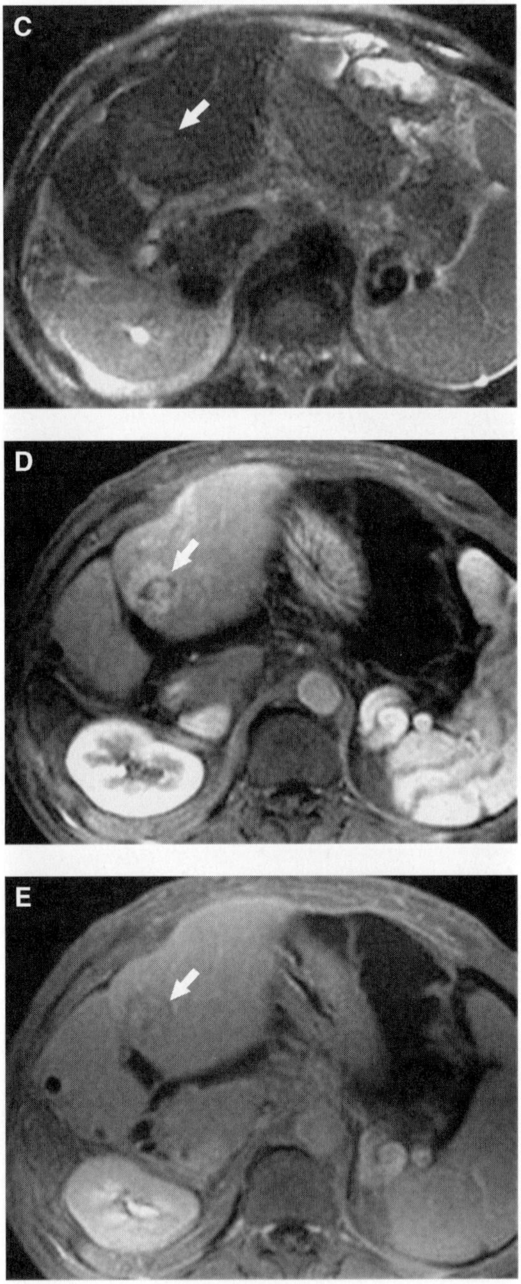


Fig. 10 (*continued*).

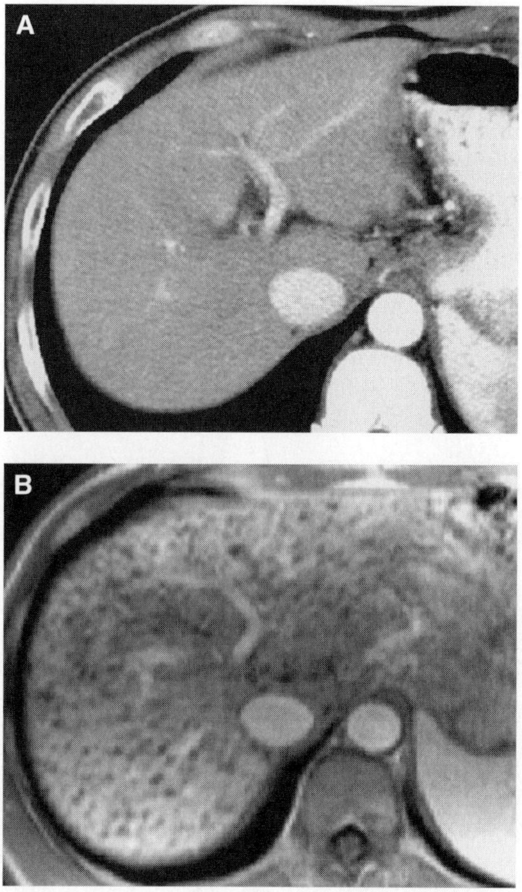


Fig. 11. Siderotic RNs. (*A*) On a portal venous phase CT scan, there is no discernible nodule in the liver. (*B*) Gradient-echo T1-weighted MR scan reveals innumerable nodules showing dark signal intensity scattered throughout the liver, indicating siderotic RNs.

DNs are usually homogeneous and show variable echogenicity on US imaging [33,34]. The occasional high echogenicity of DNs is partly explained by their fat content [35]. Signal intensity on T2-weighted MR imaging is useful for estimating the grade of malignancy of hepatocellular nodules; most DNs and some well-differentiated HCCs show isointensity or hypointensity compared with the surrounding liver parenchyma (Fig. 12), whereas almost all moderately or poorly differentiated HCCs demonstrate mild hyperintensity (Fig. 1) [33,34]. However, the signal intensity of liver nodules partly depends on the MR imaging sequences and the choice of MR scanners, and is therefore difficult to standardize. For example, the use of breath-hold T2-weighted imaging sequences based on rapid acquisition with relaxation enhancement technique tends to show

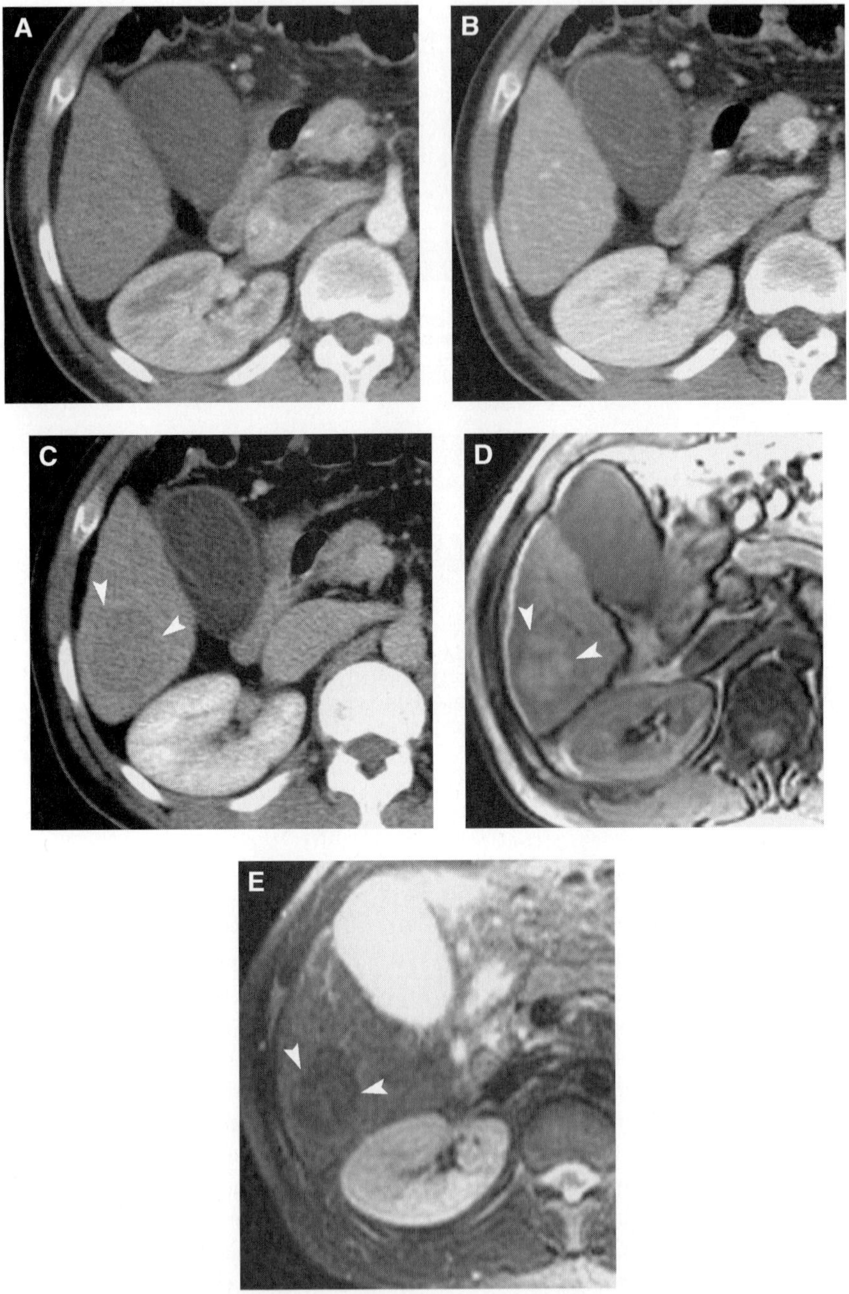
A
B
C
D
E

lower signal intensity of solid liver lesions than that obtained with nonbreath-hold spin-echo sequences. A nodule that is hyperintense on T1-weighted image and hypointense on T2-weighted image usually indicates a DN (Fig. 12) or well-differentiated HCC.

Dynamic contrast-enhanced CT or MR scan is also very useful for estimating the grade of malignancy if the AP scan is optimal. Most DNs are iso- or hypo-attenuating on arterial, portal, and delayed-phase images (Fig. 12) [33,34]; however, DNs infrequently show increased arterial vascularity [36]. On micro-bubble-enhanced US, most DNs show similar vascularity or slightly decreased vascularity compared with the adjacent liver parenchyma. Differentiation of DNs from well-differentiated HCCs is extremely difficult and sometimes not possible by imaging findings alone. A DN with a subfocus of HCC may be seen as a nodule with a focus of arterial enhancement (Fig. 13) or an isointense/hypointense nodule with a focus of hyperintensity on T2-weighted MR imaging [1].

## Mimickers of hepatocellular carcinoma in a cirrhotic liver

Nontumorous AP shunts are the most common mimickers of HCC in a cirrhotic liver. The exact mechanisms of the development of these AP shunts are not fully understood. Occlusion of small hepatic venules and retrograde filling of portal flow by way of AP anastomoses has been suggested as a cause. In addition, the formation of capillaries and the abnormal permeability of hepatic sinusoids might be also related to these lesions. The typical imaging findings of non-tumorous AP shunts include small, peripherally located, and wedge-shaped enhancing lesions seen on AP CT (Fig. 14) [5] or MR scanning [6]. These lesions never show negative enhancement compared with the adjacent liver parenchyma during the portal and delayed phases. Small HCCs associated with transtumoral AP shunts may show a similar appearance; however, the incidence of small HCCs with arterioportal shunts is not high. In fact, small hemangiomas are more frequently associated with AP shunts than are small HCCs (Fig. 15) [37,38]. Nontumorous AP shunts are generally not seen on US or unenhanced CT/MR imaging. On contrast-enhanced US, nontumorous AP shunts are infrequently visualized. However, scanning through the entire liver including the suspected area of a focal liver lesion during the portal or delayed phase is helpful to detect any portal perfusion defects in the liver.

Fig. 12. A DN. (*A–C*) Triphasic liver CT images obtained at arterial- (*A*), portal venous- (*B*), and 3-minute delayed (*C*) phases show a homogeneous, subtly hypoattenuating mass (*arrowheads*) only appreciated on a delayed phase scan (*C*). (*D–E*) The mass (*arrowheads*) shows mild hyperintensity on a T1-weighted MR scan (*D*) and mild hypointensity on a T2-weighted MR scan (*E*). The signal intensity is classic for a DN, although unusually large in size. Histopathology of resected specimen revealed low-grade DN (not shown).

Hemangioma is the most common benign tumor in the liver and potentially mimics the appearance of HCC, especially if the lesion is small. The majority of hemangiomas are seen as typical hyperechoic lesions on US, but these findings are not specific for hemangioma, as DNs or HCCs with fatty metamorphosis can show the same findings. Moreover, hemangiomas can be seen as a hypoechoic mass in a fatty liver. The enhancement features of peripheral globular enhancement with gradual central fillin on contrast-enhanced US/CT/MR imaging are virtually pathognomonic of a hemangioma. However, a hemangioma with rapid contrast enhancement may be seen as a homogeneous-enhancing nodule on both the arterial and portal phase, a pattern that is nonspecific [39]. The

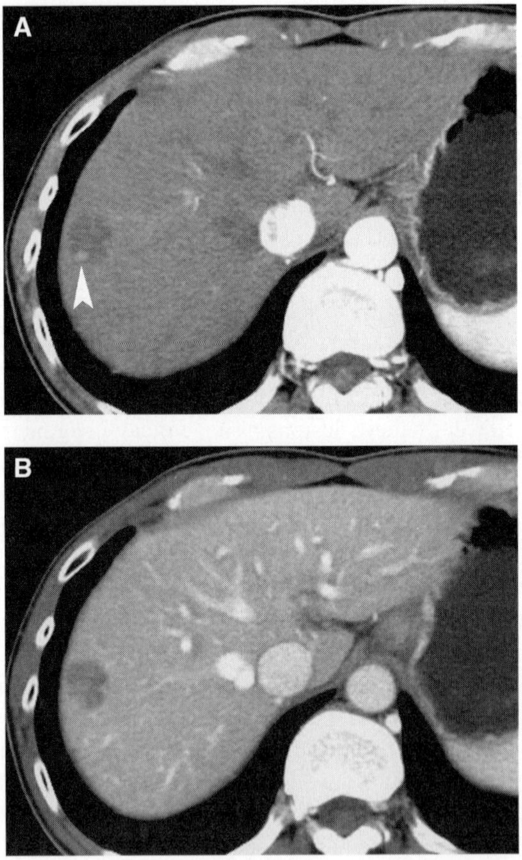


Fig. 13. Interval progression of malignant foci in the background of DN. (*A*) An AP CT scan shows a tiny hypervascular focus (*arrowhead*) in a predominantly hypoattenuating mass containing fat confirmed by MR imaging (not shown). (*B*) On a portal venous phase CT scan, the enhancing focus washes out. (*C–D*) Arterial- (*C*) and portal venous phase (*D*) CT scans obtained 9 months later shows marked interval growth of the enhancing component (*arrowhead*) largely replacing the hypoattenuating mass.

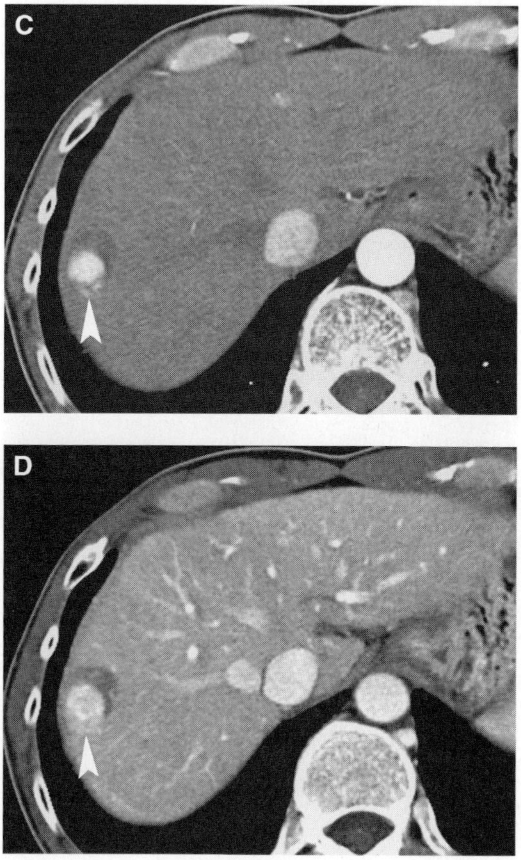


Fig. 13 (*continued*).

intensity of contrast enhancement is usually stronger in hemangioma than HCC. The presence of an AP shunt associated with a small enhancing nodule is also more suggestive of hemangioma than HCC (Fig. 15) [37]. However, the differentiation is not always clear. MR imaging can solve these problems by demonstrating typical bright hyperintensity of hemangiomas on T2-weighted imaging. Contrast-enhanced US is also extremely useful for characterization of small hemangiomas by demonstrating nodular enhancement with gradual fillin of contrast enhancement over time, regardless of the rate at which it occurs (Fig. 16) [21,39,40].

## Diagnostic accuracy of imaging tests

The diagnostic accuracy of imaging tests for HCC is extremely variable, and may strongly depend on the patient group. Most studies with patient under-

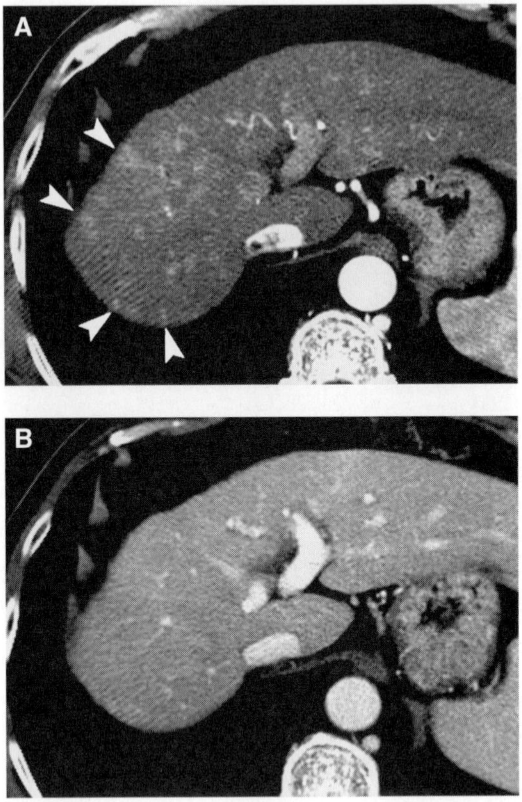

Fig. 14. Nontumorous arterioportal shunts in the cirrhotic liver. (*A*) An AP CT image shows numerous hyperattenuating foci (*arrowheads*), mostly subcapsular in location, homogeneous, and wedge-shaped, typical for arterioportal shunts. (*B*) On portal venous phase scan, all lesions become isoattenuating compared with the adjacent liver parenchyma. The lesions are stable or invisible on follow-up CT examination (not shown) obtained 15 months later.

going liver transplantation reported very low sensitivity and high specificity for detection of HCC [41–44]. The poor sensitivity might be related to advanced cirrhotic changes of the liver, which impair accurate imaging diagnosis. By comparison, many studies with patient populations having liver resection showed relatively high sensitivity for detecting HCC [45,46], probably related to the fact that the patients had relatively mild liver cirrhosis amenable to partial liver resection.

Preoperative evaluation of HCC requires a high sensitivity for the detection of any additional nodules elsewhere in the liver. Multiphasic liver CT is the most commonly used preoperative imaging modality because its sensitivity for detecting HCC is reasonably high in candidates for liver resection and CT scan is best able to evaluate extrahepatic organs. MR imaging is usually used as a problem-solving method in cases with an atypical mass or indeterminate liver

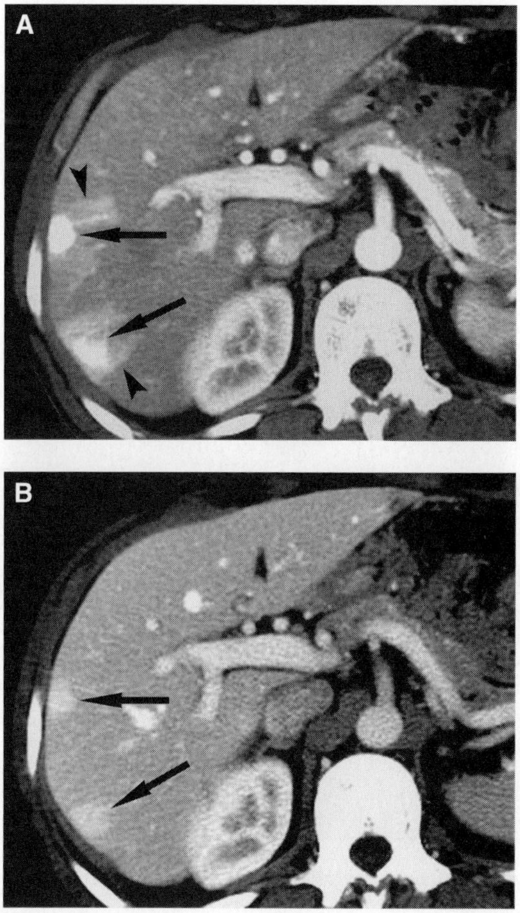


Fig. 15. Hemangiomas associated with an arterioportal shunt. (*A*) An AP CT scan shows two small nodules (*arrows*) with intense, homogeneous enhancement. Noted are wedge-shaped areas of faint enhancement (*arrowheads*) containing early opacified portal venous branches representing arterioportal shunts, associated with the intensely enhancing nodules. (*B*) On a portal venous phase scan, the nodules (*arrows*) show persistent homogeneous enhancement, consistent with hemangiomas. The areas of arterioportal shunts become isoattenuating to the parenchyma.

lesions on CT or US. MR imaging with superparamagnetic iron oxide can be a useful alternative for detecting additional liver masses, and can show higher diagnostic accuracy than multiphasic CT scan [45,46]. CT during arterial portography and CT during hepatic arteriography can be used for preoperative evaluation of HCC, and show the best sensitivity for detection of HCCs; however, the presence of frequent pseudolesions may be problematic [47]. Detailed analysis of the lesion morphology is helpful to differentiate pseudolesions from true HCCs [48,49]. These invasive CT procedures are infrequently performed because of their invasiveness.

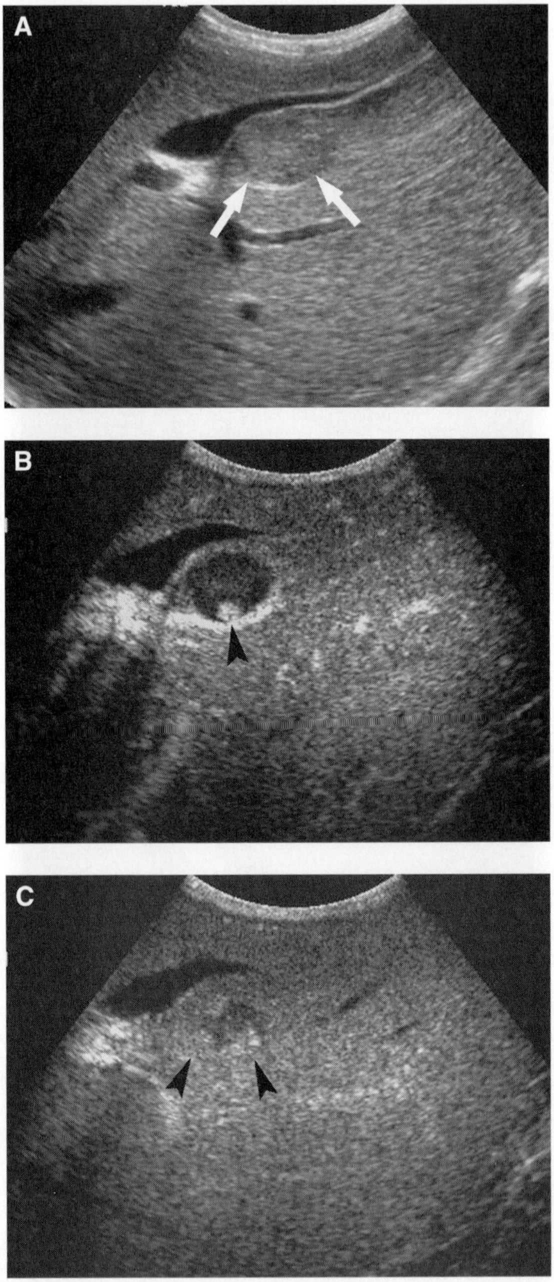


Fig. 16. Hemangioma newly detected on a surveillance US in a patient with chronic hepatitis B. (*A*) Transverse US scan shows a slightly hypoechoic nodule (*arrows*) with a bulging contour. (*B–C*) Subsequent contrast-enhanced US with microbubbles demonstrates peripheral nodular enhancement on the early phase (*B*, *arrowhead*) with central fillin pattern on the delayed phase (*C*, *arrowheads*) diagnostic of hemangioma.

US is a useful, practical, and realistic imaging test for screening HCC in high-risk patients [50,51]. The detection of small focal lesions in a cirrhotic liver requires adequate skills and experience as well as an understanding of a variety of cirrhosis-related hepatocellular nodules. The advanced cirrhotic liver, however, is often small, and may be difficult to visualize. It is also difficult to define a mass within an extremely heterogeneous liver containing numerous RNs. Therefore, contrast-enhanced CT or MR imaging can be considered for screening in selective patients with advanced liver cirrhosis with poor US scans or where there is a high clinical suspicion of HCC. Contrast-enhanced US may have a role for immediate characterization of newly detected small nodules on screening US and small indeterminate lesions seen on CT or MR scan.

## Summary

Recent advances in liver imaging techniques and better understanding of imaging findings have facilitated the detection and characterization of hepatocellular nodules in a cirrhotic liver. It is important to recognize that various types of benign nodules and pseudolesions are identified on all imaging scans performed for the diagnosis of HCC. An accurate differentiation between them is critical for adequate management of cirrhotic patients. Unfortunately, any of the imaging tests and even percutaneous biopsy are not diagnostic for borderline lesions. Intimate collaboration of hepatologists, pathologists, surgeons, and radiologists with reasonable imaging and clinical criteria estimating the degree of malignancy is imperative.

## References

[1] Choi BI, Takayasu K, Han MC. Small hepatocellular carcinomas and associated nodular lesions of the liver: pathology, pathogenesis, and imaging findings. AJR Am J Roentgenol 1993;160(6):1177–87.

[2] Sakamoto M, Hirohashi S, Shimosato Y. Early stages of multistep hepatocarcinogenesis: adenomatous hyperplasia and early hepatocellular carcinoma. Hum Pathol 1991;22(2):172–8.

[3] Freeny PC, Baron RL, Teefey SA. Hepatocellular carcinoma: reduced frequency of typical findings with dynamic contrast-enhanced CT in a non-Asian population. Radiology 1992;182(1): 143–8.

[4] Brannigan M, Burns PN, Wilson SR. Blood flow patterns in focal liver lesions at microbubble-enhanced US. Radiographics 2004;24(4):921–35.

[5] Kim TK, Choi BI, Han JK, et al. Nontumorous arterioportal shunt mimicking hypervascular tumor in cirrhotic liver: two-phase spiral CT findings. Radiology 1998;208(3):597–603.

[6] Yu JS, Kim KW, Jeong MG, et al. Nontumorous hepatic arterial-portal venous shunts: MR imaging findings. Radiology 2000;217(3):750–6.

[7] Hong SS, Kim TK, Sung KB, et al. Extrahepatic spread of hepatocellular carcinoma: a pictorial review. Eur Radiol 2003;13(4):874–82.

[8] Kim TK, Han JK, Chung JW, et al. Intraperitoneal drop metastases from hepatocellular carcinoma: CT and angiographic findings. J Comput Assist Tomogr 1996;20(4):638–42.

[9] Toyoda H, Kumada T, Kiriyama S, et al. Changes in the characteristics and survival rate of hepatocellular carcinoma from 1976 to 2000: analysis of 1365 patients in a single institution in Japan. Cancer 2004;100(11):2415–21.
[10] Matsui O, Kadoya M, Kameyama T, et al. Benign and malignant nodules in cirrhotic livers: distinction based on blood supply. Radiology 1991;178(2):493–7.
[11] Hayashi M, Matsui O, Ueda K, et al. Correlation between the blood supply and grade of malignancy of hepatocellular nodules associated with liver cirrhosis: evaluation by CT during intraarterial injection of contrast medium. AJR Am J Roentgenol 1999;172(4):969–76.
[12] Ueda K, Terada T, Nakanuma Y, et al. Vascular supply in adenomatous hyperplasia of the liver and hepatocellular carcinoma: a morphometric study. Hum Pathol 1992;23(6):619–26.
[13] Roncalli M, Roz E, Coggi G, et al. The vascular profile of regenerative and dysplastic nodules of the cirrhotic liver: implications for diagnosis and classification. Hepatology 1999;30(5):1174–8.
[14] Choi BI, Kim CW, Han MC, et al. Sonographic characteristics of small hepatocellular carcinoma. Gastrointest Radiol 1989;14(3):255–61.
[15] Tanaka S, Kitamura T, Fujita M, et al. Color Doppler flow imaging of liver tumors. AJR Am J Roentgenol 1990;154(3):509–14.
[16] Choi BI, Kim TK, Han JK, et al. Power versus conventional color Doppler sonography: comparison in the depiction of vasculature in liver tumors. Radiology 1996;200(1):55–8.
[17] Kim AY, Choi BI, Kim TK, et al. Hepatocellular carcinoma: power Doppler US with a contrast agent-preliminary results. Radiology 1998;209(1):135–40.
[18] Choi BI, Kim TK, Han JK, et al. Vascularity of hepatocellular carcinoma: assessment with contrast-enhanced second-harmonic versus conventional power Doppler US. Radiology 2000;214(2):381–6.
[19] Park SH, Kim TK, Lee KH, et al. Quantitative comparison of tumor vascularity of hepatocellular carcinoma after intravenous contrast agent: conventional versus harmonic power Doppler US. Abdom Imaging 2001;26(2):178–83.
[20] Wilson SR, Burns PN. Liver mass evaluation with ultrasound: the impact of microbubble contrast agents and pulse inversion imaging. Semin Liver Dis 2001;21(2):147–59.
[21] Kim TK, Choi BI, Han JK, et al. Hepatic tumors: contrast agent-enhancement patterns with pulse-inversion harmonic US. Radiology 2000;216(2):411–7.
[22] Kim TK, Kim AY, Choi BI. Hepatocellular carcinoma: harmonic ultrasound and contrast agent. Abdom Imaging 2002;27(2):129–38.
[23] Dill-Macky MJ, Burns PN, Khalili K, et al. Focal hepatic masses: enhancement patterns with SH U 508A and pulse-inversion US. Radiology 2002;222(1):95–102.
[24] Jang HJ, Lim HK, Lee WJ, et al. Focal hepatic lesions: evaluation with contrast-enhanced gray-scale harmonic US. Korean J Radiol 2003;4(2):91–100.
[25] Choi BI, Lee HJ, Han JK, et al. Detection of hypervascular nodular hepatocellular carcinomas: value of triphasic helical CT compared with iodized-oil CT. AJR Am J Roentgenol 1997;168(1):219–24.
[26] Hwang GJ, Kim MJ, Yoo HS, et al. Nodular hepatocellular carcinomas: detection with arterial-, portal-, and delayed-phase images at spiral CT. Radiology 1997;202(2):383–8.
[27] Choi BI, Han JK, Cho JM, et al. Characterization of focal hepatic tumors. Value of two-phase scanning with spiral computed tomography. Cancer 1995;76(12):2434–42.
[28] Lee KH, Choi BI, Han JK, et al. Nodular hepatocellular carcinoma: variation of tumor conspicuity on single-level dynamic scan and optimization of fixed delay times for two-phase helical CT. J Comput Assist Tomogr 2000;24(2):212–8.
[29] Lim JH, Choi D, Kim SH, et al. Detection of hepatocellular carcinoma: value of adding delayed phase imaging to dual-phase helical CT. AJR Am J Roentgenol 2002;179(1):67–73.
[30] Kadoya M, Matsui O, Takashima T, et al. Hepatocellular carcinoma: correlation of MR imaging and histopathologic findings. Radiology 1992;183(3):819–25.
[31] Pauleit D, Textor J, Bachmann R, et al. Hepatocellular carcinoma: detection with gadolinium- and ferumoxides-enhanced MR imaging of the liver. Radiology 2002;222(1):73–80.

[32] International Working Party. Terminology of nodular hepatocellular lesions. Hepatology 1995; 22(3):983–93.
[33] Choi BI, Han JK, Hong SH, et al. Dysplastic nodules of the liver: imaging findings. Abdom Imaging 1999;24(3):250–7.
[34] Lim JH, Choi BI. Dysplastic nodules in liver cirrhosis: imaging. Abdom Imaging 2002;27(2): 117–28.
[35] Kim MJ, Lim JH, Lee SJ, et al. Correlation between the echogenicity of dysplastic nodules and their histopathologically determined fat content. J Ultrasound Med 2003;22(4):327–34.
[36] Lim JH, Cho JM, Kim EY, et al. Dysplastic nodules in liver cirrhosis: evaluation of hemodynamics with CT during arterial portography and CT hepatic arteriography. Radiology 2000;214(3):869–74.
[37] Byun JH, Kim TK, Lee CW, et al. Arterioportal shunt: prevalence in small hemangiomas versus that in hepatocellular carcinomas 3 cm or smaller at two-phase helical CT. Radiology 2004;232(2):354–60.
[38] Kim KW, Kim TK, Han JK, et al. Hepatic hemangiomas with arterioportal shunt: findings at two-phase CT. Radiology 2001;219(3):707–11.
[39] Jang HJ, Kim TK, Lim HK, et al. Hepatic hemangioma: atypical appearances on CT, MR imaging, and sonography. AJR Am J Roentgenol 2003;180(1):135–41.
[40] Kim JH, Kim TK, Kim BS, et al. Enhancement of hepatic hemangiomas with levovist on coded harmonic angiographic ultrasonography. J Ultrasound Med 2002;21(2):141–8.
[41] Lim JH, Park CK. Hepatocellular carcinoma in advanced liver cirrhosis: CT detection in transplant patients. Abdom Imaging 2004;29(2):203–7.
[42] Liu WC, Lim JH, Park CK, et al. Poor sensitivity of sonography in detection of hepatocellular carcinoma in advanced liver cirrhosis: accuracy of pretransplantation sonography in 118 patients. Eur Radiol 2003;13(7):1693–8.
[43] Peterson MS, Baron RL, Marsh Jr JW, et al. Pretransplantation surveillance for possible hepatocellular carcinoma in patients with cirrhosis: epidemiology and CT-based tumor detection rate in 430 cases with surgical pathologic correlation. Radiology 2000;217(3):743–9.
[44] Krinsky GA, Lee VS, Theise ND, et al. Transplantation for hepatocellular carcinoma and cirrhosis: sensitivity of magnetic resonance imaging. Liver Transpl 2002;8(12):1156–64.
[45] Kang BK, Lim JH, Kim SH, et al. Preoperative depiction of hepatocellular carcinoma: ferumoxides-enhanced MR imaging versus triple-phase helical CT. Radiology 2003;226(1): 79–85.
[46] Kim SK, Kim SH, Lee WJ, et al. Preoperative detection of hepatocellular carcinoma: ferumoxides-enhanced versus mangafodipir trisodium-enhanced MR imaging. AJR Am J Roentgenol 2002;179(3):741–50.
[47] Jang HJ, Lim JH, Lee SJ, et al. Hepatocellular carcinoma: are combined CT during arterial portography and CT hepatic arteriography in addition to triple-phase helical CT all necessary for preoperative evaluation? Radiology 2000;215(2):373–80.
[48] Kim HC, Kim TK, Sung KB, et al. Preoperative evaluation of hepatocellular carcinoma: combined use of CT with arterial portography and hepatic arteriography. AJR Am J Roentgenol 2003;180(6):1593–9.
[49] Kim HC, Kim TK, Sung KB, et al. CT during hepatic arteriography and portography: an illustrative review. Radiographics 2002;22(5):1041–51.
[50] Mima S, Sekiya C, Kanagawa H, et al. Mass screening for hepatocellular carcinoma: experience in Hokkaido, Japan. J Gastroenterol Hepatol 1994;9(4):361–5.
[51] Nguyen MH, Keeffe EB. Screening for hepatocellular carcinoma. J Clin Gastroenterol 2002; 35(5 suppl 2):86–91.

ELSEVIER
SAUNDERS

Clin Liver Dis 9 (2005) 281–285

CLINICS IN
LIVER DISEASE

# Liver Biopsy in the Diagnosis of Hepatocellular Carcinoma

Ian R. Wanless, MD, FRCPC

*Department of Pathology, The Toronto Hospital, 200 Elizabeth Street, Toronto, Canada, M5G 2C4*

Modern imaging techniques have allowed the discovery of many small and asymptomatic hepatic lesions that pose a new challenge to pathologists. These lesions are difficult to diagnose histologically because small lesions tend to be well differentiated, with subtle deviations from normal. Pathologists outside of referral centers do not have comprehensive experience with these lesions.

## Classification and nomenclature

Study of resected hepatocellular carcinoma (HCC) reveals a high prevalence of small premalignant lesions in the same liver [1,2]. These lesions have atypical features that distinguish them from normal or cirrhotic liver but are not sufficient for the diagnosis of carcinoma. They are thought to be premalignant because small regions of carcinoma can often be found within these otherwise benign lesions. Individual investigators have applied different names to these lesions, including macroregenerative nodules, adenomatous hyperplasia, and dysplastic nodules. The International Working Party of the World Congresses of Gastroenterology recommended consolidation of the nomenclature to “dysplastic nodule” [3].

## Presentation

Moderately differentiated hepatocellular carcinomas are usually hypervascular with enhancement on modalities that detect arterial flow [4]. Early malignant lesions may be isovascular or hypovascular, and become hypervascular upon

*E-mail address:* ian.wanless@utoronto.ca

1089-3261/05/$ – see front matter 
doi:10.1016/j.cld.2004.12.005 *liver.theclinics.com*

Table 1
IWP histologic criteria to distinguish hepatocellular nodules

| Histologic feature | Large regenerative nodule | Dysplastic nodule, low grade | Dysplastic nodule, high grade | Well-differentiated HCC | Moderately differentiated HCC |
|---|---|---|---|---|---|
| Clone-like populations | – | + | + | + | + |
| Plates more than 3 cells wide | – | – | – | – | + |
| Mitotic figures > 5/10 HPF | – | – | – | – | + |
| Cell density more than twice normal[a] | – | – | – | + | + |
| Invasion of stroma or portal tracts | – | – | – | + | + |
| Irregular nuclear contour, at least moderate | – | – | – | + | + |
| Absence of portal tracts (arterial supply) | – | – | +/– | + | + |
| Mitotic figures, occasional (1–5/10 HPF)[c] | – | – | + | + | + |
| Cell density more than 1.3 times normal | – | – | + | + | + |
| Nuclear hyperchromasia | – | – | + | + | + |
| Irregular nuclear contour, at least mild | – | – | + | + | + |
| Pseudogland formation | +[b] | – | + | + | + |
| Cytoplasmic basophilia | | – | + | + | + |
| Cytoplasmic clear cell change | – | – | + | + | + |
| Reticulin less than normal | – | – | – | – | + |
| Increased or decreased iron accumulation | – | + | + | + | + |

*Abbreviations*: IWP, International Working Party; HCC, hepatocellular carcinoma; HPF, high power field (10 × 40).

[a] As a measure of increased nuclear to cytoplasmic ratio.

[b] Especially when cholestasis present.

[c] Mitoses may occur in any lesion in the presence of cholestasis or recent necrosis.

*Data from* Wanless IR for the International Working Party. Terminology of nodular hepatocellular lesions. Hepatology 1995;22:983–93.

further growth. The portal vein supply is lost as arteries grow to supply the growing lesion. This is reflected on CT with arterioportography as a negative tumor blush during the portal venous phase. A third of early carcinomas has abundant steatosis [5].

## Pathology

The pathologist recognizes dysplastic nodules only when the size or texture differs from the background cirrhotic nodules. This generally occurs when the nodule reaches 5 mm, although for study purposes a cutoff of 10 mm has often been used. Generally, nodules greater than 1.5 cm achieve histologic criteria of HCC. However, occasionally, benign dysplastic nodules may reach a 2-cm diameter without definite malignant transformation. Aspiration cytology can be used for a reliable diagnosis of moderately differentiated HCC, but tissue sections are usually required for dysplastic nodules and well-differentiated carcinoma.

The histologic features listed in Table 1 may assist in the diagnosis. Carcinoma is suggested by hepatocellular plates more than two cells in thickness. Reticulin, trichrome, or periodic acid schiff stains facilitate this assessment. Well-differentiated HCC may have single or double plates so that other criteria must be considered. Atypical architectural features including pseudoglandular forms, and double plates with deviation of the nuclei to the sinusoidal margins are suggestive of HCC. An increased nucleus-to-cytoplasmic ratio is particularly useful. HCC should have some nuclear atypia, although this is often mild.

Invasion of stroma is a useful criterion for malignancy [6,7]. However, biopsy samples seldom have this feature. There are a number of look-alike conditions where benign and nonneoplastic hepatocytes migrate into stromal areas as well as lumina of portal and hepatic veins. Therefore, this criterion should not be accepted unless there are supportive cytologic and architectural features of carcinoma. Mitotic figures are not helpful to diagnose well-differentiated HCC. Loss of reticulin may occur, especially in moderately differentiated HCC. Immunohistochemical stain for CD34 or CD31 highlights the arterial supply of a nodule; endothelial cells that line arterialized sinusoidal stain positively [8]. Although this staining is more prominent in HCC, it also occurs focally in dysplastic nodules and benign cirrhotic nodules. The hepatocytes of most HCCs are positive for glipican-3, but focal and weak staining limits its diagnostic usefulness [9].

Dysplastic nodules may be low grade or high grade. Low-grade dysplastic nodules are not suggestive of malignancy, and high-grade dysplastic nodules have atypical features but not sufficient criteria for the diagnosis of HCC. Low-grade dysplastic nodules are difficult to distinguish from regenerative nodules because of the minimal nuclear atypia and normal nucleus/cytoplasmic (N/C) ratio in both conditions. The most useful feature is the presence of map-like areas of uniform cellular appearance especially in background cirrhotic nodules. Small clusters less than 1 mm in diameter of atypical hepatocytes have been defined as dysplastic foci. These are most often recognized as iron-free foci in patients with hemochromatosis [10].

Regenerative nodules in nonneoplastic conditions may resemble dysplastic nodules or HCC [11]. This is particularly the case in fulminant hepatic failure, severe cholestasis, and Budd-Chiari syndrome when regenerative stimuli are extreme. These regenerative nodules often have mitoses, widened plates, moderate increase in N/C ratio, and active nuclear chromatin pattern. Regenerative nodules are supplied by portal tracts, often with ductular proliferation. Clinical history is important to avoid these difficulties.

Adenoma may be difficult to distinguish from well-differentiated HCC [11]. The history of exposure to oral contraceptives or anabolic steroids may be comforting. However, HCC can also occur in this clinical setting. Shrinkage of the lesion on cessation of the medication is one of the best diagnostic criteria for adenoma. A lesion many centimeters in diameter that has minimal abnormalities of nuclei, N/C ratio, and plate structure is usually benign. Generally adenoma does not have mitoses, and the plates are uniform and no more than two cells in thickness.

Focal nodular hyperplasia can usually be diagnosed when there is a central scar, a regular arrangement of arteries, and periarterial connective tissue containing ductal elements [11]. There is a newly recognized form of adenoma in which portal elements may be found. This has been called telangiectatic hepatocellular adenoma as well as "telangiectatic focal nodular hyperplasia" [12]. Nonhepatocellular lesions such as angiomyolipoma may be distinguished by negative heppar-1 (hepatocyte, Dako) and Cam5.2 stains.

## Interobserver variation

The International Consensus Group for Hepatic Neoplasia is currently assessing the reliability of histologic diagnosis of early HCC and dysplastic nodules. This group of two dozen hepatopathologists from 10 countries met in 2002 and 2004. The results of these meetings will be published in detail elsewhere. The results indicated considerable variation in diagnoses rendered for a study set of resected lesions. It was evident that refinements of the diagnostic criteria and a teaching aid for general pathologists was needed. A new diagnostic approach is being developed, to be known as the Laennec Classification of Hepatocellular Neoplasia.

## The Laennec Classification of Hepatic Neoplasia

The proceedings of the The International Consensus Group for Hepatic Neoplasia indicated that there were many histologic criteria that were difficult to apply because of subjective assessment. Furthermore, some criteria were of value only in large resection specimens; a lower grade of neoplasia was often diagnosed in a biopsy from the same lesion. The proposed Laennec Classification of Hepatocellular Neoplasia system will be defined in detail elsewhere. The system can be applied to premalignant lesions and all grades of hepatocellular carcinoma.

In this system, nuclear atypia, N/C ratio, and architectural atypia are graded 0–4 or 0–6 with the assistance of a standard set of photographs. The scores of these three components are summed, giving a possible range of 0–14. When two or more distinct regions are noted, more than one Laennec score is reported along with a comment on the percentage of the lesion occupied by each score. Stromal invasion, mitoses, and arterialization are not considered in this system because they are highly dependent on sample size.

The advantages of this system are (1) it can be applied to both small and large samples, (2) complexity is reduced, (3) criteria are standardized, and (4) the use of a numerical score reinforces the fact that early neoplastic features form a spectrum. The clinical significance of a given Laennec score is currently being evaluated.

## References

[1] Wada K, Kondo F, Kondo Y. Large regenerative nodules and dysplastic nodules in cirrhotic livers: a histopathologic study. Hepatology 1988;8:1684–8.

[2] Theise ND, Park YN, Kojiro M. Dysplastic nodules and hepatocarcinogenesis. Clin Liver Dis 2002;6:497–512.

[3] Wanless IR for the International Working Party. Terminology of nodular hepatocellular lesions. Hepatology 1995;22:983–93.

[4] Sakabe K, Yamamoto T, Kubo S, et al. Correlation between dynamic computed tomographic and histopathological findings in the diagnosis of small hepatocellular carcinoma. Dig Surg 2004; 21:413–20.

[5] Kutami R, Nakashima Y, Nakashima O, et al. Pathomorphologic study on the mechanism of fatty change in small hepatocellular carcinoma of humans. J Hepatol 2000;33:282–9.

[6] Kondo F, Kondo Y, Nagato Y, et al. Interstitial tumour cell invasion in small hepatocellular carcinoma. Evaluation in microscopic and low magnification views. J Gastroenterol Hepatol 1994;9:604–12.

[7] Nakano M, Saito A, Yamamoto M, et al. Stromal and blood vessel wall invasion in well-differentiated hepatocellular carcinoma. Liver 1997;17:41–6.

[8] Roncalli M, Roz E, Coggi G, et al. The vascular profile of regenerative and dysplastic nodules of the cirrhotic liver: implications for diagnosis and classification. Hepatology 1999;30:1174–8.

[9] Capurro M, Wanless IR, Sherman M, et al. Related Glypican-3: a novel serum and histochemical marker for hepatocellular carcinoma. Gastroenterology 2003;125:89–97.

[10] Deugnier YM, Charalambous P, Le Quilleuc D, et al. Preneoplastic significance of hepatic iron-free foci in genetic hemochromatosis: a study of 185 patients. Hepatology 1993;18:1363–9.

[11] Wanless IR. Benign liver tumors. Clin Liver Dis 2002;6:513–26.

[12] Paradis V, Benzekri A, Dargere D, et al. Telangiectatic focal nodular hyperplasia: a variant of hepatocellular adenoma. Gastroenterology 2004;126:1323–9.

ELSEVIER
SAUNDERS

Clin Liver Dis 9 (2005) 287–300

CLINICS IN
LIVER DISEASE

# Chemoembolization and Bland Embolization: A Critical Appraisal

Alex S. Befeler, MD

*Division of Gastroenterology and Hepatology, Saint Louis University, 3635 Vista @ Grand FDT 9S, St. Louis, MO 63110, USA*

Hepatocellular carcinoma (HCC) is a major cause of cancer-related mortality worldwide, resulting in more than 500,000 deaths per year [1]. In the West, HCC is becoming the most frequent cause of liver-related death in patients with viral-associated cirrhosis [2]. In the United States, the incidence of HCC increased 114% between 1975 and 1998, with the fastest growing age group in recent years being those 45 to 55 years old [3]. Unfortunately, only about 30% of the patients diagnosed with HCC in surveillance programs are candidates for potentially curative therapy such as liver transplantation, surgical resection, or local ablation [4]. Without surveillance only 10% to 15% of patients are eligible for potentially curative treatment.

Palliative therapy includes options such as bland embolization, chemoembolization, and chemotherapy (intraarterial and systemic). Chemotherapy has only limited utility in HCC because of poor objective response rates (generally less than 25%) and lack of survival benefit [5,6]. Thus, chemotherapy should be offered in the setting of clinical investigation of new agents for patients with advanced stage disease [6]. Those patients with intermediate-stage disease (tumors either too large or multicentric for curative treatment and relatively preserved hepatic function) are candidates for embolization therapy [5,6]. There have been seven randomized clinical trials [7–13] comparing embolization treatment to supportive care or ineffective treatment and four systematic reviews/meta-analyses [14–17]. This article will critically evaluate the various roles for bland and chemoembolization of HCC.

*E-mail address:* befelera@slu.edu


doi:10.1016/j.cld.2004.12.011

## How does embolization therapy work?

The goal of embolization therapy is to disrupt the blood supply to HCC while limiting collateral damage to the nontumorous liver. In the case of chemoembolization, there is the additional delivery of a high concentration of chemotherapeutic agents that remain in contact with the lesion for a prolonged period of time. The rationale supporting the technique comes from the observation that >90% of the blood supply to HCC comes from the hepatic artery where about 80% of the blood supply to the normal liver comes from the portal vein [18]. In theory, the embolization causes ischemia of the tumor, and combined with chemotherapy, result in tumor necrosis. Greater than 95% tumor necrosis is seen on pathologic examination in 70% of small HCC after a single bland embolization, but only 44% for lager tumors [19]. The chemotherapy is usually mixed with iodized poppy seed oil (lipiodol) forming an emulsion that traps the chemotherapy and tends to concentrate in HCC [20]. The concentration of chemotherapy in the tumor may be 10 to 100 times greater than if given systemically [21]. Additionally, the embolization induces tumor ischemia, which blocks transmemebrane pumps and directly limits the chemotherapy from washing out of the tumor cells [20]. Despite these observations, the true mechanism of producing tumor necrosis remains unknown [20].

## Technique

There are local variations in the techniques of embolization therapy. Generally, the patient enters the angiography suite following an overnight fast. After volume loading with normal saline, administration of sedatives and prophylactic antibiotics (not all centers give prophylaxis), a visceral angiogram is performed to identify the arterial anatomy of the liver, the size and locations of the tumors, and their feeding vessels and portal venous potency. A catheter is advanced beyond the gastroduodenal artery (to avoid extrahepatic embolization), and depending on tumor location to lobar, segmental, or subsegmental branches feeding the target lesion(s). Chemotherapy, in combination with lipiodol (for chemoembolization), and embolization materials (gelatin sponges) such as Gelfoam (Pharmacia and Upjohn, Kalamazoo, Michigan) or Ivalon (M-PACT Worldwide Inc., Eudora, Kansas) or polyvinyl alcohol particles are injected sequentially [20]. The gelatin sponges cause only temporary thrombosis lasting about 2 weeks, whereas polyvinyl alcohol is more permanent [20]. Patients are admitted for continued volume loading, antibiotics, and pain management for 24 to 48 hours [22].

The choice of chemotherapeutic agents used with embolization generally includes cisplatin [8,10,13], doxorubicin [11,12], and epirubicin [23,24]. Two studies compared doxorubicin to epirubicin and found no differences in overall survival [24,25]. Doxorubicin was compared with cisplatin in nonrandomized studies, with two showing improved overall survival with cisplatin [26,27] and one showing no differences [28]. In addition, one of the strongly positive randomized controlled trials (RCTs) assessing chemoembolization therapy used doxorubicin [11] and the other used cisplatin [10]. Thus, there is no convincing evidence that one agent is better than another, and an RCT comparing doxorubicin to cisplatin is warranted.

The dose of chemotherapeutic agents for chemoembolization varies among centers. Chen et al demonstrated in a randomized trial that for Child A patients high-dose lipiodol chemoembolization (epirubicin 50 $mg \cdot m^{-2}$, mitomycin C 8 $mg \cdot m^{-2}$, and iodized oil mean dose 28 mL) sometimes followed by resection resulted in better survival compared with a standard dose [29]. No differences in survival were found by another group who assessed conventional (mitomycin C 10 mg, epirubicin 40 mg, and carboplatin 300 mg) versus low-dose (mitomycin C 2–8 mg, epirubicin 0–10 mg, carboplatin 0–100 mg based upon tumor diameter) lipiodol chemoembolization in a nonrandomized study [30].

Most centers repeat chemoembolization based upon response assessed by imaging, hepatic reserve, and a planned interval usually every 2 to 4 months [9–11,13]. One nonrandomized study suggested improved survival with repeated treatments based upon response and hepatic reserve alone [31].

## Complications

The most common toxicity (32–80%) from embolization therapy is a self-limited postembolization syndrome consisting of fever, abdominal pain, vomiting, and sometimes elevations in alanine aminotransferase (ALT) [8,10,13,32]. Postprocedural pain may be limited by administration of lidocaine during the procedure [33,34]. Other complications occurring in generally $<10\%$ of cases include new or worsening ascites, gastrointestinal bleeding from varices or ulcers, leukopenia, and worsening hepatic function [8,10,11,13,32]. Rare but significant complications include death, cholecystitis, ischemic hepatitis, liver abscess, bacteremia, hepatic failure, and renal failure [11,13,35]. Persistent renal failure is associated with Child-Pugh class B and diabetes mellitus [35]. Long-term oral supplementation with branched chain amino acids resulted in significant improvements in postchemoembolization albumin, bilirubin, and quality of life, reduced complications including ascites and edema, but no effects on survival [36].

## Efficacy for primary treatment of hepatocellular carcinoma

The "gold standard" to assess the efficacy of any therapy is to rely on the results of large RCTs comparing treatment to no treatment in a well-defined and uniform group of patients [15,37]. No large RCTs are available for embolization therapy, but the literature contains seven smaller RCTs [7–13]. Meta-analysis is generally considered the next best level of proof of efficacy, and combines the results of several smaller RCTs to usually overcome the lack of statistical power of individual studies [15,37]. It relies upon uniformity of the combined trials with regard to treatments and patient populations. Even if the combined trials have adequate statistical uniformity, meta-analyses may disagree with large RCTs 10% to 23% of the time [37]. Many nonrandomized trials, some with controls, are available to assess the efficacy of embolization therapy, but without randomization there are bound to be significant biases, which are likely to have a major impact on the end point assessed.

Efficacy of treatment for HCC should be defined by survival differences rather than tumor-free survival or objective tumor responses because of the generally high mortality. In these patients, survival is clearly dependent upon both tumor progression and hepatic failure [5]. Although some therapies may effectively treat the tumor, the collateral damage to the liver may result in shortened survival due to liver failure. Additionally, because even with therapy the mortality remains high, quality of life should be part of the assessment of treatment. Thus, embolization therapy is generally limited to patients who are not candidates for curative therapy and who are thought to have adequate reserve to undergo the procedure.

Llovet et al [38] studied the natural history of a group of patients with these characteristics who were randomized to no treatment arms of two clinical trials. They showed that performance status, constitutional syndrome (weight loss, malaise, and anorexia), invasion of the portal vein, and extrahepatic spread of tumor were independent predictors of mortality [38]. Presence of any one of these parameters changed 1-, 2-, and 3-year survival from 80%, 65%, and 50%, respectively, to 29%, 16%, and 8% [38]. Another study of a similar group of untreated patients with HCC found that the presence of a variant estrogen receptor transcript and bilirubin levels were the best predictors of survival [39]. They found 1-, 2-, and 3-year survival of 94%, 66%, and 52% with the wild-type estrogen receptor, and 51%, 21%, and 16% with the variant estrogen receptor, respectively [39]. Although these predictors of survival need further validation, the magnitude of their apparent effects is much larger than any of the results from the RCTs of embolization therapy. Other factors such as Child-Pugh score, tumor morphology, $\alpha$-fetoprotein level, and portal vein thrombosis, which make up the Cancer Liver Italian Program and Okuda staging systems, are also predictive of survival in treated patients with HCC [40,41]. Clearly, with and without treatment many factors relating to both the tumor and the underlying liver disease can drastically alter the survival of patients with HCC. Thus, only randomized trials should be relied upon for overall assessment of embolization therapies.

Additionally, differences in treatment protocols including number of cycles and addition of chemotherapeutic agents may alter outcomes. There may also be interaction between the effects of embolization treatment and the amount of hepatic reserve where patients with limited hepatic reserve may have worse survival with treatment and those with more reserve may have better survival.

A careful examination of these issues will help explain the differences in the outcomes of the RCTs for embolic therapy. Llovet et al [15] performed a meta-analysis of seven RCTs including 545 patients assessing primary treatment of HCC not amendable to potentially curative treatment. Bland embolization or chemoembolization were compared with no treatment or ineffective treatment (tamoxifen or intravenous 5-fluorouracil) as a control [15]. There was a significant improvement in 2-year survival (odds ratio [OR], 0.53, 95% confidence interval [CI], 0.32–0.89) in the six trials that reported 2-year results (Fig. 1) [15]. The missing trial [12] had 22% of patients with end-stage disease, Okuda III, compared with none in the other trials. When all seven trials were assessed for 1-year survival there was only trend toward favoring treatment (OR, 0.64, 95% CI, 0.41–1.01) [15]. Sensitivity analysis showed significant benefit of treatment versus no treatment, treatment for the five high-quality trials, and chemoembolization versus control, but no benefit of embolization versus control (Fig. 2) [15]. The strength of Llovet et al's [14,16,17] analysis over all the previous analyses is inclusion of all the available RCTs published to date. The analysis shows a strong suggestion of benefit for chemoembolization.

So why were three of the studies clearly negative [9,12,13] and two clearly positive [10,11]? Statistical testing for heterogeneity between the trials was negative, but the patient populations differed substantially, with 1- and 2-year survival in the control groups ranging from 13% to 80% and 11% to 50%, respectively. The control group survival in the positive Western study [11] was

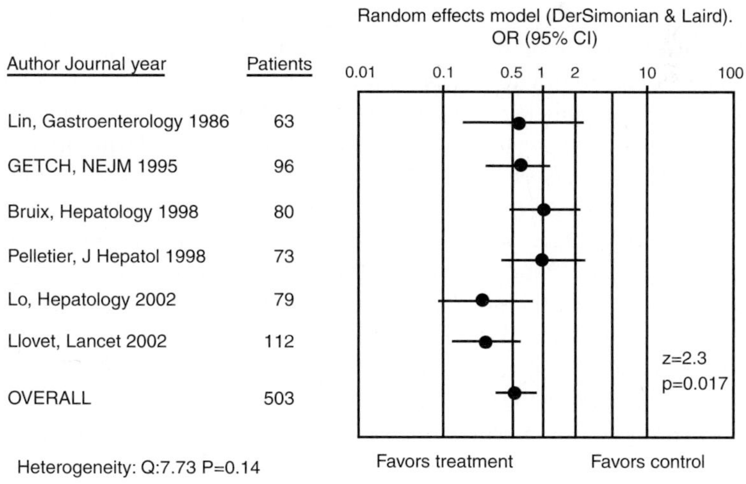


Fig. 1. Meta-analysis of RCTs comparing embolization therapy versus consevvative or ineffective treatments. Random effects model (OR, 0.53; 95% CI, 0.32–0.89; $P = 0.017$. (*From* Llovet J, Bruix J. Systematic review of randomized trials for unresectable hepatocellular carcinoma: chemoembolization improves survival. Hepatol 2003;37:429–42. Copyright ©2003 The American Association for the Study of Liver Diseases; reprinted with permission from Wiley-Liss, Inc., a subsidiary of John Wiley & Sons, Inc.)

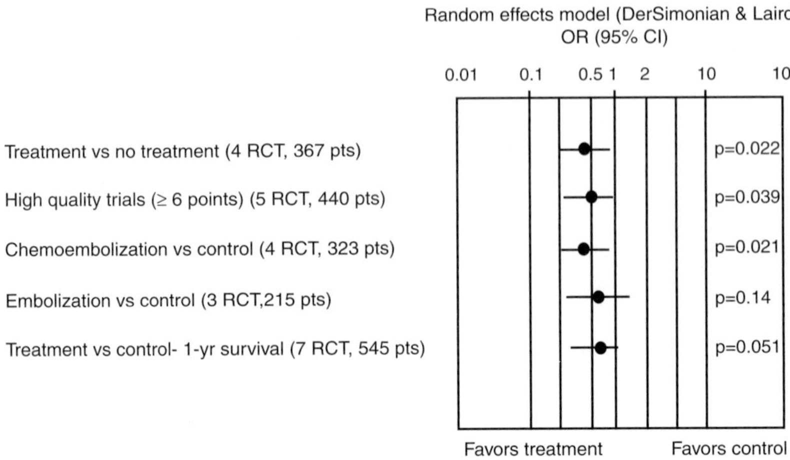


Fig. 2. Sensitivity meta-analysis of 6 RCTs reporting 2-year survival assessing embolization therapy versus conservative therapy (four RCTs), embolization therapy versus conservative or suboptimal therapy in high-quality trials (five RCTs), chemoembolization versus conservative or suboptimal therapy (four RCTs), bland embolization versus conservative or suboptimal therapy (three RCTs) ,and embolization therapy versus conservative or suboptimal therapy 1-year survival (7RCTs). (*From* Llovet J, Bruix J. Systematic review of randomized trials for unresectable hepatocellular carcinoma: chemoembolization improves survival. Hepatology 2003;37:429–42. Copyright; 2003. The American Association for the Study of Liver Diseases; reprinted with permission from Wiley-Liss, Inc., a subsidiary of John Wiley & Sons, Inc.)

among the best, whereas in the Asian trial [10] it was among the worst. These two trials generally differ from the rest by being more recent, and thus have better catheter technology to achieve more selective embolization of the tumors, using doses of chemotherapy based upon tumor size or hepatic function, using lipiodol, and repeating treatments in responders as long as hepatic function did not deteriorate. The Asian study had more advanced tumors with 25% with portal vein branch thrombosis, which probably explains their low control group survival rate [10]. There was no evidence that the patients with portal vein thrombosis benefited from treatment [10]. All the negative studies lacked at least one of these factors—selective embolization [7,8,12,13], chemoembolization [7,9], dose adjustment for chemotherapy [8,12], repeated treatments [9], and repeated treatments based upon tumor response or liver function [8,12].

Repeated chemoembolization and bland versus chemoembolization have been assessed carefully in other trials. A sequential nonrandomized assessment of every 2-month repeated chemoembolization versus retreatment based upon response found better survival with the latter [42]. The choice between bland embolization and chemoembolization is controversial. There are two RCTs comparing bland to chemoembolization from the 1980s and early 1990s that showed no survival differences between the therapies [43,44]. The most recent meta-analysis of embolization therapy versus control found that chemoembolization and not bland embolization improves survival [15]. Only one of the studies [11] made a direct comparison that showed no statistical difference in survival between chemoembolization and bland embolization, but the study was underpowered to compare the procedures. It found a definite survival benefit for chemoembolization, and suggested a possible benefit of bland embolization. Thus, the evidence supporting a benefit for chemoembolization therapy is stronger than bland embolization.

## Predictors of survival

Multiple studies have tried to assess predictors of survival in patients undergoing embolization therapy. Predictors of survival include unilobar portal vein thrombosis, performance status, ascites, bilirubin, $\alpha$-fetoprotein, Child-Pugh class, Cancer Liver Italian Program score, Model for End-Stage Liver Disease score, and tumor size [8,10,45–48]. Exact cutoffs for the predictors are not readily available, and even some patients with poor predictors can achieve 5-year survivals [48]. Most centers, including those that performed the two positive RCTs, suggest not treating patients with main or lobar portal vein thrombosis, Okuda III, poor performance status, and extrahepatic disease [5,10,11]. There are limitations of these studies, because without a large RCT, it is difficult to separate independent predictors of survival that should relate to the underlying liver disease, tumor biology, the treatment and interaction between all these factors.

## Efficacy before surgical resection

The data regarding the efficacy of embolization therapy before planned resection of HCC is limited by being predominately retrospective and sometimes relying upon disease-free survival rather than the more valid overall survival. Embolization therapy before resection is performed to prevent long-term recurrence of tumor, and sometimes to downstage a previously unresectable tumor. There are two Asian RCTs that attempt to prevent recurrence of tumor by preoperative embolization. The first compares preoperative chemoembolization versus direct resection in 52 patients with tumors >10 cm and generally preserved hepatic function (50% noncirrhotic) [49]. It showed worse overall survival with chemoembolization [49]. The study results may have been compromised because the chemoembolization group had a much higher rate of invasion of adjacent organs, although the high rate may have been a result of the mean 18-week delay to surgery while getting chemoembolization [49]. The second compares preoperative bland embolization versus direct resection in 97 patients with tumors 3 cm to 5 cm, and showed no difference in cancer-free or overall survival [50]. The remaining studies in the literature are retrospective, nonrandomized, with only one [51] with a carefully matched control. It included 48 patients with mean tumor size 7.8 cm, and showed no differences in cancer-free or overall survival [51]. Recent large series with no overall survival or tumor-free survival benefits included 889 Asian [52–57] and 76 Western patients [58] with generally large tumors. Three of the series [54,55,57] suggested that large or advanced tumors did receive a survival benefit, and one [58] suggested that 10% of previously unresectable patients were downstaged by chemoembolization. Di Carlo et al showed overall survival benefit compared with control in a group of 100 patients with tumors <5 cm [59]. Gerunda et al showed improved tumor-free but not over all survival in 40 patients with mean 4-cm tumors [60]. Many chemoembolization patients never made it to resection and were excluded, thus negating the conclusions [60]. Overall, there is no convincing evidence to recommend preresection chemoembolization. A randomized controlled trial of chemoembolization pre-resection for patients with large tumors including potentially unresectable tumors in patients with preserved hepatic function would be welcome, but these patients are rare in North America.

## Efficacy before orthotopic liver transplantation

Orthotopic liver transplantation (OLT) is a highly effective treatment for HCC because it provides the widest possible resection margins and replaces the damaged liver [5]. By following the Milan criteria (solitary lesion <5 cm or two to three lesions each <3 cm and no extra hepatic spread or vascular invasion) [61], multiple series have demonstrated >70% long-term survival for patients with HCC treated by OLT, which is nearly identical to outcomes in patients without HCC [61–64]. These excellent results occurred at a time when mean waiting times were <6 months [38]. Unfortunately, the dropout rate for patients with HCC on OLT waiting lists can exceed 20% [65,66]. Thus, intention to survival is markedly reduced because nearly all of the dropouts have very poor survival.

Graziadei et al [67] showed that chemoembolization in patients meeting the Milan criteria while waiting for OLT could eliminate waiting list dropouts and produce 5-year survival rates of 94% despite a waiting time of a mean of 178 days (range 28–459). Harnois et al [68] evaluated a similar chemo-embolization protocol including patients with up to three HCC nodules each <5 cm. The pre-OLT drop out rate was 7%, with a waiting time of a mean of 167 days (range 28–548). Survival in those transplanted was 84% at 2 years despite having 37% of the patients exceeding the Milan criteria, and there was no recurrence of HCC [68]. A longer term assessment of pre-OLT chemo-embolization from the same group involving many of the same patients showed a cumulative probability of dropout due to a tumor progression of 15% at 6 months and 25% at 12 months [69]. Post-OLT 5-year survival was 74%, but it decreased to 61% if assessed by intention-to-treat analysis [69].

Complications resulting in lost opportunity to proceed with transplant or death from pre-OLT chemoembolization are rare [67–69]. Posttransplant complications also appear to be rare [67–69], and one series addressing the issue of hepatic artery complications did not show increased rates compared with other OLT patients [70]. Thus, chemoembolization may have a role in controlling HCC while a patient is waiting for OLT especially if the waiting time is likely to be 6 or more months. There does not appear to be a significant detrimental effect of chemoembolization on these patients provided that they have adequate hepatic reserve. Chemoembolization has not been compared with other options such as ethanol or radiofrequency ablation in this setting. Fortunately for patients with HCC in the United States, pre-OLT treatments may be unnecessary given the currently short waiting times with the special exception listing for HCC in the Model for End-Stage Liver Disease organ allocation system. Thirty- and 90-day transplantation rates are 26% and 44% for <2 cm lesions and 47% and 76%, respectively, for other lesions meeting the Milan criteria [71]. The criteria were recently changed to giving additional advantage only to patients with the larger or multiple tumors, but waiting times should continue to remain low [72].

Some have proposed expanding the Milan criteria to permit OLT in more patients with HCC [25,67,73]. Chemoembolization may be able to downstage these patients. Roayaire et al [25] assessed 80 patients with tumors >5 cm who underwent attempted downstaging. They were unable to downstage 46%, but the remaining who went on to OLT had a survival of 44% at 5 years [25]. The decreased survival compared with the >70% long-term survival found in other series was generally due to tumor recurrence, and could be reduced by restricting transplant to tumors <7 cm and without vascular invasion [25]. Another group performed a similar assessment of chemoembolization for advanced tumors and had a 27% dropout rate and a 41% 4-year survival [67]. Thus, overall intention-to-treat survivals in these patients are poor, but some patients appear to have long-term benefit. Downstaging with chemoembolization before OLT should be limited to research protocols attempting to find predictors of better long-term success.

## Efficacy in combination with local ablative therapy

Percutaneous ethanol ablation is a standard treatment for small HCC [5]. Combination of chemoembolization followed by ethanol ablation for tumors <3 cm compared with chemoembolization alone has been evaluated and found not to significantly affect long-term survival, but may reduce recurrence [74,75]. Similar therapy for large tumors assessed by nonrandomized comparisons suggested improved long-term survival [76–78]. A randomized trial of chemoembolization plus local ablative therapy versus chemoembolization alone is warranted.

## Summary

Bland embolization and chemoembolization are commonly used therapies for patients with HCC who are not candidates for curative treatment. Thus, their role is palliative, and should be applied to patients with larger or multiple tumors who have sufficient hepatic reserve. The ability of chemoembolization as primary treatment to prolong survival has recently been demonstrated by meta-analysis. The evidence for efficacy of bland embolization is weaker. The role of embolization therapy before resection or OLT is controversial, and warrants assessment by RCT.

## References

[1] Parkin DM, Bray F, Ferlay J, et al. Estimating the world cancer burden: Globocan 2000. Int J Cancer 2001;94:153–6.
[2] Benvegnù L, Gios M, Boccato S, et al. Natural history of compensated viral cirrhosis: a prospective study on the incidence and hierarchy of major complication. Gut 2004;53: 744–9.
[3] El-Serag H, Davila J, Petersen N, et al. The continuing increase in the incidence of hepatocellular carcinoma in the United States: an update. Ann Intern Med 2003;139(10):817–23.
[4] Llovet J, Burroughs A, Bruix J. Hepatocellular carcinoma. Lancet 2003;362:1907–17.
[5] Befeler A, Di Bisceglie A. Hepatocellular carcinoma: diagnosis and treatment. Gastroenterology 2002;122:1609–19.
[6] Llovet J, Brú C, Bruix J. Prognosis of hepatocellular carcinoma: the BCLC staging classification. Semin Liver Dis 1999;19(3):329–38.
[7] Lin D, Liaw Y, Lee T, et al. Hepatic arterial embolization in patients with unresectable hepatocellular carcinoma—a randomized controlled trial. Gastroenterology 1988;94:453–6.
[8] Anonymous. A comparison of lipiodol chemoembolization and conservative treatment for unresectable hepatocellular carcinoma. N Engl J Med 1995;332(19):1256–61.
[9] Bruix J, Llovet JM, Castells A, et al. Transarterial embolization versus symptomatic treatment in patients with advanced hepatocellular carcinoma: results of a randomized, controlled trial in a single institution. Hepatology 1998;27:1578–83.
[10] Lo C, Ngan H, Tso W, et al. Randomized controlled trial of transarterial lipiodol chemoembolization for unresectable hepatocellular carcinoma. Hepatology 2002;35:1164–71.
[11] Llovet JM, Real MI, Montañá X, et al. Arterial embolisation or chemoembolisation versus symptomatic treatment in patients with unresectable hepatocellular carcinoma: a randomized controlled trial. Lancet 2002;359:1734–9.
[12] Pelletier G, Roche A, Ink O, et al. A randomized trial of hepatic arterial chemoembolization in patients with unresectable hepatocellular carcinoma. J Hepatol 1990;11(2):181–4.
[13] Pelletier G, Ducreaux M, Gay F, et al. Treatment of unresectable hepatocellular carcinoma with lipidol chemoembolization: a multicenter randomized trial. J Hepatol 1998;29:129–34.
[14] Camma C, Schepis F, Orlando A, et al. Transarterial chemoembolization for unresectable hepatocellular carcinoma: meta-analysis of randomized controlled trials. Radiology 2002; 224(1):47–54.
[15] Llovet J, Bruix J. Systematic review of randomized trials for unresectable hepatocellular carcinoma: chemoembolization improves survival. Hepatology 2003;37:429–42.
[16] Mathurin P, Rixe O, Carbonell N, et al. Overview of medical treatments in unresectable hepatocellular carcinoma—an impossible meta-analysis? Aliment Pharmacol Ther 1998;12: 111–26.

[17] Simonetti RG, Liberati A, Angiolini C, et al. Treatment of hepatocellular carcinoma: a systematic review of randomized controlled trials. Ann Oncol 1997;8(2):117–36.
[18] Breedis C, Young G. The blood supply of neoplasm of the liver. Am J Pathol 1954;30: 969–85.
[19] Higuchi T, Kikuchi M, Okazaki M. Hepatocellular carcinoma after transcatheter hepatic arterial embolization: a histopathologic study of 84 resected cases. Cancer 1994;73(9):2259–67.
[20] Ramsey D, Kernagis L, Soulen M, et al. Chemoembolization of hepatocellular carcinoma. J Vasc Interv Radiol 2002;13:S211–21.
[21] Konno T. Targeting cancer chemotherapeutic agents by use of lipiodol contrast medium. Cancer 1990;66:1897–903.
[22] Poon RT, Ngan H, Lo C, et al. Transarterial chemoembolization for inoperable hepatocellular carcinoma and postresection intrahepatic recurrence. J Surg Oncol 2000;73:109–14.
[23] Kawai S, Tani M, Okamura J, et al. Prospective and randomized trial of lipiodol-transcatheter arterial chemoembolization for treatment of hepatocellular carcinoma: a comparison of epirubicin and doxorubicin (second cooperative study). Semin Oncol 1997;24(2 suppl 6): S6-38–45.
[24] Watanabe S, Nishioka M, Ohta Y, et al. Prospective and randomized controlled study of chemoembolization therapy in patients with advanced hepatocellular carcinoma. Cancer Chemother Pharmacol 1994;33(suppl):S93–6.
[25] Roayaie S, Frischer J, Emre S, et al. Long-term results with multimodal adjuvant therapy and liver transplantation for the treatment of hepatocellular carcinomas larger than 5 centimeters. Ann Surg 2002;235(4):533–9.
[26] Ono Y, Yoshimasu T, Ashikaga R, et al. Long-term results of lipiodol-transcatheter arterial embolization with cisplatin or doxorubicin for unresectable hepatocellular carcinoma. Am J Clin Oncol 2000;23(6):564–8.
[27] Kamada K, Nakanishi T, Kitamoto M, et al. Long-term prognosis of patients undergoing transcatheter arterial chemoembolization for unresectable hepatocellular carcinoma: comparison of cisplatin lipiodol suspension and doxorubicin hydrochloride emulsion. J Vasc Interv Radiol 2001;12:847–54.
[28] Uenoi K, Miyazono N, Inoue H, et al. Transcatheter arterial chemoembolization therapy using iodized oil for patients with unresectable hepatocellular carcinoma: evaluation of three kinds of regimens and analysis of prognostic factors. Cancer 2001;88(7):1574–81.
[29] Chen MS, Li JQ, Zhang YQ, et al. High-dose iodized oil transcatheter arterial chemoembolization for patients with large hepatocellular carcinoma. World J Gastroenterol 2002; 8(1):74–8.
[30] Lu W, Li Y, He X, et al. Transcatheter arterial chemoembolization for hepatocellular carcinoma in patients with cirrhosis: evaluation of two kinds of dosages of anticancer drugs and analysis of prognostic factors. Hepatogastroenterology 2003;50(54):2079–83.
[31] Ernst O, Sergent G, Mizrahi D, et al. Treatment of hepatocellular carcinoma by transcatheter arterial chemoembolization: comparison of planned periodic chemoembolization and chemoembolization based on tumor response. AJR Am J Roentgenol 1999;172(1):59–64.
[32] Chan A, Yuen MF, Hui CK, et al. A prospective study regarding the complications of transcatheter intraarterial lipiodol chemoembolization in patients with hepatocellular carcinoma. Cancer 2002;94(6):1747–52.
[33] Lee SH, Hath ST, Park SH. Intraarterial lidocaine administration for relief of pain resulting from transarterial chemoembolization of hepatocellular carcinoma: its effectiveness and optimal timing of administration. Cardiovas Interven Radiol 2001;24(6):368–71.
[34] Romano M, Giojelli A, Tamburrini O, et al. Chemoembolization for hepatocellular carcinoma: effect of intraarterial lidocaine in peri- and post-procedural pain and hospitalization. Radiol Med (Torino) 2003;105(4):350–5.
[35] Huo TI, Wu JC, Huang YH, et al. Acute renal failure after transarterial chemoembolization for hepatocellular carcinoma: a retrospective study of the incidence, risk factors, clinical course and long-term outcome. Aliment Pharmacol Ther 2004;19(9):999–1007.
[36] Poon R, Yu W-C, Fan S-T, et al. Long-term oral branched chain amino acids in patients

undergoing chemoembolization for hepatocellular carcinoma: a randomized trial. Aliment Pharm Ther 2004;19:779–88.
[37] Ioannidis J, Cappelleri J, Lau J. Issues in comparisons between meta-analyses and large trials. JAMA 1998;279(14):1089–93.
[38] Llovet J, Bustamante J, Castells A, et al. Natural history of untreated nonsurgical hepatocellular carcinoma: rationale for the design and evaluation of therapeutic trials. Hepatology 1999;29(1):62–7.
[39] Villa E, Moles A, Ferretti I, et al. Natural history of inoperable hepatocellular carcinoma: estrogen receptors' status in the tumor is the strongest prognostic factor for survival. Hepatology 2000;32(2):233–8.
[40] CLIP Investigators. Prospective validation of the CLIP score: a new prognostic system for patients with cirrhosis and hepatocellular carcinoma. Hepatology 2000;31(4):840–5.
[41] Okuda K, Ohtsuki T, Obata H, et al. Natural history of hepatocellular carcinoma and prognosis in relation to treatment: study of 850 patients. Cancer 1995;56:918–28.
[42] Ernst O, Sergent G, Mizrahi D, et al. Treatment of hepatocellular carcinoma by transcatheter arterial chemoembolization: comparison of planned periodic chemoembolization and chemoembolization based on tumor response. AJR Am J Roentgenol 1999;172:59–64.
[43] Chang JM, Tzeng WS, Pan HB, et al. Transcatheter arterial embolization with or without cisplatin treatment of hepatocellular carcinoma: a randomized controlled study. Cancer 1994;74(9):2449–53.
[44] Kawai S, Okamura J, Ogawa M, et al. Prospective and randomized clinical trial for the treatment of hepatocellular carcinoma—a comparison of lipiodol-transcatheter arterial embolization with and without adriamycin (first cooperative study). Cancer Chemotherapy & Phamacol 1992;31(Suppl):S1–6.
[45] Testa R, Testa E, Giannini E, et al. Trans-catheter arterial chemobolisation for hepatocellular carcinoma in patients with viral cirrhosis: role of combined staging systems, Cancer Liver Italian Program (CLIP) and Model for End-stage Liver Disease (MELD), in predicting outcome after treatment. Aliment Pharmacol Ther 2003;17:1563–9.
[46] Lladó L, Virgili J, Figueras J, et al. A prognostic index of the survival of patients with unresectable hepatocellular carcinoma after transcatheter arterial chemoembolization. Cancer 2000;88(1):50–7.
[47] Mondazzi L, Bottelli R, Brambilla G, et al. Transarterial oily chemoembolization for the treatment of hepatocellular carcinoma: a multivariate analysis of prognostic factors. Hepatol 1994;19(5):1115–23.
[48] O'Suilleabhain CB, Poon RTP, Young J, et al. Factors predictive of 5-year survival after transarterial chemoembolization for inoperable hepatocellular carcinoma. Br J Surg 2003; 90:325–31.
[49] Wu C-C, Ho Y-Z, Ho W, et al. Preoperative transcatheter arterial chemoembolization for resectable large hepatocellular carcinoma: a reappraisal. Br J Surg 1995;82(1):122–6.
[50] Yamasaki S, Hasegawa H, Kinoshita H, et al. A prospective randomized trial of the preventive effect of preoperative transcatheter arterial embolization against recurrence of hepatocellular carcinoma. Jpn J Cancer Res 1996;87(2):206–11.
[51] Paye F, Jagot P, Vilgrain V, et al. Preoperative chemoembolization of hepatocellular carcinoma: a comparative study. Arch Surg 1998;133(7):767–72.
[52] Uchida M, Kohno H, Kubota H, et al. Role of preoperative transcatheter arterial oily chemoembolization for resectable hepatocellular carcinoma. World J Surg 1996;20:326–31.
[53] Harada T, Matsuo K, Inoue T, et al. Is pre-operative hepatic arterial chemoembolization safe and effective for hepatocellular carcinoma? Ann Surg 1996;224(1):4–9.
[54] Lu CD, Peng SY, Jiang XC, et al. Preoperative transcatheter arterial chemoembolization and prognosis of patients with hepatocellular carcinoma: retrospective analysis of 120 cases. World J Surg 1999;23:293–300.
[55] Luo YQ, Wang Y, Chen H, et al. Influence of preoperative transcatheter arterial chemoembolization on liver resection in patients with resectable hepatocellular carcinoma. Hepatobiliary Pancreat Dis Int 2002;1(4):523–6.

[56] Ochiai T, Sonoyama T, Hironaka T, et al. Hepatectomy with chemoembolization for treatment of hepatocellular carcinoma. Hepatogastroenterology 2003;50(51):750–5.
[57] Sugo H, Futagawa S, Beppu T, et al. Role of preoperative transcatheter arterial chemoembolization for resectable hepatocellular carcinoma: relation between postoperative course and the pattern of tumor recurrence. World J Surg 2003;27:1295–9.
[58] Majno PE, Adam R, Bismuth H, et al. Influence of preoperative transarterial lipiodol chemoembolization on resection and transplantation for hepatocellular carcinoma in patients with cirrhosis. Ann Surg 1997;226(6):688–703.
[59] Di Carlo V, Ferrari G, Castoldi R, et al. Pre-operative chemoembolization of hepatocellular carcinoma in cirrhotic patients. Hepatogastroenterology 1998;45(24):1950–4.
[60] Gerunda GE, Neri D, Merenda R, et al. Role of transarterial chemoembolization before liver resection for hepatocarcinoma. Liver Transpl 2000;6(5):619–26.
[61] Mazzaferro V, Regalia E, Doci R, et al. Liver transplantation for the treatment of small hepatocellular carcinomas in patients with cirrhosis. N Engl J Med 1996;334:693–9.
[62] Figueras J, Jaurrieta E, Valls C, et al. Survival after liver transplantation in cirrhotic patients with and without hepatocellular carcinoma: a comparative study. Hepatology 1997;25:1485–9.
[63] Bismuth H, Majno P, Adam R. Liver transplantation for hepatocellular carcinoma. Semin Liver Dis 1999;19:311–28.
[64] Llovet JM, Bruix J, Fuster J, et al. Liver transplantation for small hepatocellular carcinoma: the tumor-node-metastasis classification does not have prognostic power. Hepatology 1998;27: 1572–7.
[65] Llovet JM, Fuster J, Bruix J. Intention-to-treat analysis of surgical treatment for early hepatocellular carcinoma: resection versus transplantation. Hepatology 1999;30:1434–40.
[66] Yao FY, Bass NM, Nikolai B, et al. A follow-up analysis of the pattern and predictors of dropout from the waiting list for liver transplantation in patients with hepatocellular carcinoma: implications for current organ allocation policy. Liver Transpl 2002;9(7):684–92.
[67] Graziadei I, Sandmueller K, Waldenberger P, et al. Chemoembolization followed by liver transplantation for hepatocellular carcinoma impedes tumor progression while on the waiting list and leads to excellent outcome. Liver Transpl 2003;9(6):557–63.
[68] Harnois D, Steers J, Andrews J, et al. Preoperative hepatic artery chemoembolization followed by orthotopic liver transplantation for hepatocellular carcinoma. Liver Transpl Surg 1999; 5(3):192–9.
[69] Maddala Y, Stadheim L, Andrews J, et al. Drop-out rates of patients with hepatocellular cancer listed for liver transplantation: outcome with chemoembolization. Liver Transpl 2004; 10(3):449–55.
[70] Richard III HM, Silberzweig JE, Mitty HA, et al. Hepatic arterial complications in liver transplant recipients treated with pretransplantation chemoembolization for hepatocellular carcinoma. Radiology 2000;214(3):775–9.
[71] Freeman RB, Wiesner RH, Roberts JP, et al. 2003 SRTR report on the state of transplantation: improving liver allocation: MELD and PELD. Am J Transpl 2004;4(suppl 9):114–31.
[72] United Network for Organ Sharing Policy 3.6. www.unos.org/policiesandbylaws/policies.asp. Accessed September 14, 2004.
[73] Yao F, Ferrell L, Bass N, et al. Liver transplantation for hepatocellular carcinoma: expansion of the tumor size limits does not adversely impact survival. Hepatology 2001;33(6):1394–403.
[74] Kamada K, Kitamoto M, Aikata H, et al. Combination of transcatheter arterial chemoembolization using cisplatin-lipiodol suspension and percutaneous ethanol injection for treatment of advanced small hepatocellular carcinoma. Am J Surg 2002;184(3):284–90.
[75] Koda M, Murawaki Y, Mitsuda A, et al. Combination therapy with transcatheter arterial chemoembolization and percutaneous ethanol injection compared with percutaneous ethanol injection alone for patients with small hepatocellular carcinoma. Cancer 2001;92(6):1516–24.
[76] Lencioni R, Paolicchi A, Moretti M, et al. Combined transcatheter arterial chemoembolization and percutaneous ethanol injection for the treatment of large hepatocellular carcinoma: local therapeutic effect and long-term survival rate. Eur Radiol 1998;8(3):439–44.
[77] Yamamoto K, Masuzawa M, Kato M, et al. Evaluation of combined therapy with

chemoembolization and ethanol injection for advanced hepatocellular carcinoma. Semin Oncol 1997;24(2 suppl 6):S6–55.
[78] Dohmen K, Shirahama M, Shigematsu H, et al. Transcatheter arterial chemoembolization therapy combined with percutaneous ethanol injection for unresectable large hepatocellular carcinoma: an evaluation of the local therapeutic effect and survival rate. Hepatogastrology 2001;48(41):1409–15.

ELSEVIER
SAUNDERS

CLINICS IN
LIVER DISEASE

Clin Liver Dis 9 (2005) 301–314

# A Critical Appraisal of the Literature on Local Ablative Therapies for Hepatocellular Carcinoma

Riccardo Lencioni, MD*, Laura Crocetti, MD

*Division of Diagnostic and Interventional Radiology, Department of Oncology, Transplants, and Advanced Technologies in Medicine, University of Pisa, Via Roma 67, Pisa I-56125, Italy*

Image-guided percutaneous techniques for local tumor ablation have been one of the major advances in the treatment of hepatocellular carcinoma (HCC). Over the past 2 decades, several methods for chemical or thermal tumor destruction have been developed and clinically tested (Box 1). Percutaneous ablation techniques are currently accepted as the best therapeutic choice for patients with early-stage HCC—as defined by the Barcelona Clinic Liver Cancer staging classification [1,2]—when liver transplantation or surgical resection are not suitable options [3,4]. However, local ablative therapies share some common problems with regard to interpretation of the literature [5]. A large portion of the published research lacks either relevance or sufficient methodologic rigor to be reliable enough to help establish the beneficial and harmful effects of each procedure. Any deficiency is not predominantly in the quality of the basic research; the deficiency lies more in the lack of a general recognition that it is necessary to go beyond the case series format to establish higher levels of evidence before new techniques come into clinical practice [6]. The present article reviews the reported results of percutaneous ablation

* Corresponding author.
*E-mail address:* lencioni@do.med.unipi.it (R. Lencioni).

1089-3261/05/$ – see front matter 
doi:10.1016/j.cld.2004.12.002

**Box 1. Local ablative therapies for hepatocellular carcinoma**

Chemical ablation
- Ethanol injection
- Acetic acid injection
- Hot saline injection

Thermal ablation
- Radiofrequency ablation
- Microwave ablation
- Laser ablation

techniques in the treatment of HCC with the aim to appraise their clinical efficacy.

## Chemical ablation

### *Ethanol injection*

Percutaneous ethanol injection (PEI) has been the first and most widely used technique for local ablation of expanding, nodular-type HCC [7–9]. Ethanol induces coagulation necrosis as a result of cellular dehydration, protein denaturation, and chemical occlusion of small tumor vessels. Histopathologic studies have shown that PEI may lead to complete ablation of about 70% of tumors smaller than 3 cm in diameter [10]. PEI is best administered by using ultrasound guidance because ultrasound allows for continuous real-time monitoring of the injection. This is crucial to realize the pattern of tumor perfusion and to avoid excessive ethanol leakage outside the lesion. Fine noncutting needles, with either a single end hole or multiple side holes, are commonly used for PEI. PEI is usually performed under local anesthesia, and does not require patient hospitalization. The treatment schedule includes four to six sessions performed once or twice weekly. The number of treatment sessions, as well as the amount of injected ethanol per session, may vary greatly according to the size of the lesion, the pattern of tumor perfusion, and the compliance of the patient.

Although there have not been any prospective randomized trials comparing PEI and best supportive care or PEI and surgical resection, several retrospective studies have provided indirect evidence that PEI improves the natural history of HCC: the long-term outcomes of patients with early-stage tumors who were treated with PEI were similar to those reported in surgical series, with 5-year survival rates ranging fro 41% to 53% in Child A patients (Table 1) [11–18]. In

Table 1
Studies reporting long-term survival outcomes of patients with early-stage hepatocellular carcinoma who underwent percutaneous ethanol injection

| | | Survival rates (%) | | |
|---|---|---|---|---|
| Author and year | No. patients | 1 year | 3 years | 5 years |
| Shiina et al, 1993 [11] | 98 | 85 | 62 | 52 |
| Lencioni et al, 1995 [12] | 105 | 96 | 68 | 32 |
| Livraghi et al, 1995 [13] | | | | |
| Child A, single HCC <5 cm | 293 | 98 | 79 | 47 |
| Child B, single HCC <5 cm | 149 | 93 | 63 | 29 |
| Ryu et al, 1997 [14] | | | | |
| Stage I, 1–3 HCC <3 cm[a] | 110 | 98 | 84 | 54 |
| Stage II, 1–3 HCC <3 cm[a] | 140 | 91 | 65 | 45 |
| Lencioni et al, 1997 [15] | | | | |
| Child A, 1 HCC <5 cm or 3 <3 cm | 127 | 98 | 79 | 53 |
| Child B, 1 HCC <5 cm or 3 <3 cm | 57 | 88 | 50 | 28 |
| Pompili et al, 2001 [16] | | | | |
| Child A, 1–2 HCC <5 cm | 111 | 94 | 62 | 41 |
| Teratani et al, 2002 [17] | | | | |
| Age <70 years | 516 | 90 | 65 | 40 |
| Age >70 years | 137 | 83 | 52 | 27 |

*Abbreviation:* HCC, hepatocellular carcinoma.

[a] Clinical stage according to the Liver Cancer Study Group of Japan, Primary liver Cancer in Japan. Ann Surg 1990;221:277–87.

a retrospective comparative study including 391 patients with uninodular HCC smaller than 5 cm, the cumulative 3-year survival after surgical resection, PEI, or no treatment was 79%, 71%, and 26%, respectively, for Child A patients ($P < 0.001$ for surgery versus no treatment, $P < 0.001$ for PEI versus no treatment); and 40%, 41%, and 13%, respectively, for Child B patients ($P < 0.01$ for surgery versus no treatment, $P < 0.001$ for PEI versus no treatment), suggesting that surgery and PEI improve survival in small uninodular HCC associated with Child A or B cirrhosis compared with untreated patients in the same Child class [19]. Of importance, two cohort studies and one retrospective case–control study comparing surgical resection and PEI failed to identify any difference in survival, despite patients in PEI groups who had worse liver function (Table 2) [20–22]. These data showed that PEI is a useful treatment for patients with early-stage HCC, and suggested that surgical resection may achieve better results only after strict candidate selection.

Despite the fact that PEI is a low-risk procedure, severe complications have been reported. In a multicenter survey including 1066 patients (8118 PEI sessions), one death (0.1%) and 34 complications (3.2%)—including seven cases of tumor seeding (0.7%)—were reported [23]. The major limitation of PEI is the high local recurrence rate, that may reach 33% in lesions smaller than 3 cm and 43% in lesions exceeding 3 cm [24,25]. The injected ethanol does not always accomplish complete tumor necrosis because of its inhomogeneous distribution within the lesion—especially in the presence of intratumoral septa—

Table 2
Studies comparing surgical resection and percutaneous ethanol injection in the treatment of early-stage hepatocellular carcinoma

| | | Survival rates (%) | | | |
|---|---|---|---|---|---|
| Author and year | No. patients | 1-yr | 3-yr | 5-yr | *P* |
| Castells et al, 1993 [20][a] | | | | | NS |
| Surgical resection | 33 | 81 | 44 | NA | |
| Ethanol Injection | 30 | 83 | 55 | NA | |
| Yamamoto et al, 2001 [21][a] | | | | | NS |
| Surgical resection | 58 | 97 | 84 | 61 | |
| Ethanol Injection | 39 | 100 | 82 | 59 | |
| Daniele et al, 2003 [22][b] | | | | | NS |
| Surgical resection | 17 | 82 | 63 | NA | |
| Ethanol Injection | 65 | 91 | 65 | NA | |

*Abbreviations:* NA, not available; NS, not significant.
[a] Cohort study.
[b] Retrospective case–control study.

and the limited effect on extracapsular cancerous spread. Also, PEI is unable to create a safety margin of ablation in the liver parenchyma surrounding the nodule, and therefore may not destroy tiny satellite nodules that, even in small tumors, may be located in close proximity of the main lesion [26].

Injection of large volumes of ethanol in a single session performed under general anesthesia has been reported to increase the success rate of PEI in the treatment of large or infiltrating HCC. In a series of patients with either single, large, encapsulated HCC (n = 24, group A) or infiltrating or multiple HCC (n = 63, group B), the 1-, 2-, 3-, and 4-year survival rates were 72%, 65%, 57%, and 44%, respectively, for group A; and 73%, 60%, 42%, and 18%, respectively, for group B [27]. The authors concluded that single-session PEI may be an option for selected patients with advanced disease previously excluded from surgical treatment. However, results of single-session PEI are based on uncontrolled investigations and when critically compared with recent data about the natural history and prognosis of untreated nonsurgical HCC the benefits of the procedure are not evident. In fact, an analysis of the natural history of cirrhotic patients with HCC who were not treated within prospective randomized controlled trials reported 1-, 2-, and 3-year survival rates of 80%, 65%, and 50%, respectively, for patients with preserved performance status and absence of a constitutional syndrome, vascular invasion, or extrahepatic tumor spread [28].

### *Acetic acid and hot saline injection*

Acetic acid and hot saline injection have been proposed as viable alternatives to PEI for the treatment of HCC [29,30]. Two studies compared acetic acid injection and PEI. In the first paper, 60 patients with one to four HCC lesions smaller than 3 cm were entered into a randomized trial. The 1- and 2-year survival rates were 100% and 92%, respectively, in the acetic acid injection group; and 83% and 63%, respectively, in the PEI group ($P = 0.0017$). A multivariate analysis of prognostic factors showed that treatment was an independent predictor of survival [31]. In contrast, in a prospective comparative study including 63 patients treated by acetic acid injection and 62 patients treated by PEI, no significant survival differences were observed between the two treatment groups. The 1- and 3-year survival rates were 84% and 51%, respectively, for the acetic acid group; and 81% and 46%, respectively, for the PEI group ($P = 0.651$) [32]. The only study on survival outcomes of HCC patients receiving hot saline injection reported a median survival of 10 months (range, 3–36 months) achieved in 29 patients with a mean tumor diameter of 7 cm [33]. In summary, these alternate options for chemical ablation were used by very few investigators worldwide and were not tested in large series of patients. The reported survival outcomes are not better than those obtained by several authors with PEI.

## Thermal ablation

### *Radiofrequency ablation*

The goal of radiofrequency (RF) ablation is to induce thermal injury to the tissue through electromagnetic energy deposition. The patient is part of a closed-loop circuit that includes an RF generator, an electrode needle, and a large dispersive electrode (ground pads). An alternating electric field is created within the tissue of the patient. Because of the relatively high electrical resistance of tissue in comparison with the metal electrodes, there is marked agitation of the ions present in the target tissue that surrounds the electrode, because the tissue ions attempt to follow the changes in direction of alternating electric current. The agitation results in frictional heat around the electrode. The discrepancy between the small surface area of the needle electrode and the large area of the ground pads causes the generated heat to be focused and concentrated around the needle electrode [34].

In the initial experience with RF treatment, a major limitation the technique was the small volume of ablation created by conventional monopolar electrodes. These devices were capable of producing cylindrical ablation zones no greater than 1.6 cm in the short axis [35]. Therefore, multiple electrode insertions were necessary to treat all but the smallest lesions. Subsequently, several strategies for increasing the ablation zone achieved with RF treatment have been used. Major progress was achieved with the introduction of modified electrodes, including internally cooled electrodes [36] and multitined expandable electrodes [37]. Internally cooled electrodes consist of dual-lumen electrodes with an exposed active tip of variable length. Internal cooling is obtained by continuous perfusion with chilled saline, and is aimed at preventing overheating of tissues nearest to the electrode to minimize carbonization and gas formation around the tip [38]. Multitined expandable electrodes have an active surface that can be substantially increased by prongs deployed from the tip. In application, the tip of the needle is advanced to the target lesion and the curved electrodes are deployed into the tumor according to the desired volume of ablation [39].

RF ablation requires the use of conscious sedation or general anesthesia. Although ultrasound is considered in most centers as the preferred imaging guidance, the choice is largely dependent on the operator's expertise as well as on the availability of dedicated equipment such as computed tomography (CT) fluoroscopy or open magnetic resonance (MR) systems [40]. The treatment protocol depends on the RF system and the desired volume of ablation [41]. At the end of the procedure, the needle track can be ablated to prevent any tumor cell dissemination. The procedure is performed under standard cardiac, pressure, and oxygen monitoring.

RF ablation has been the most widely assessed alternative to PEI for local ablation of HCC. Most early clinical research with RF ablation was conducted in the framework of feasibility studies [42–44]. These investigations had merit in showing the efficacy and the safety of the procedure. However, the data were heterogeneous and unsystematically presented [45]. Moreover, RF treatment was not compared with any established treatment for HCC. The European Associaton for the Study of the Liver has recommended that newer methods of tumor destruction, such as RF ablation should be compared with the well-established and accepted PEI through randomized trials [3]. In fact, methodologic research has given convincing evidence that less rigorous study designs are likely to produce biased results and to exaggerate the estimated effect of a new therapy.

One randomized study compared RF ablation versus PEI for the treatment of early-stage HCC [46]. In this trial, 104 Child A or B patients with 144 HCC lesions (uninodular tumor <5 cm or as many as three tumors <3 cm each) were randomly assigned to receive RF ablation or PEI. No statistically significant differences between RF ablation and PEI groups were observed with respect to baseline characteristics, except for patient's age and albumin concentration. At the time of the analysis, the mean follow-up was 22 months. The overall survival rates at 1 and 2 years were 100% and 98%, respectively, in the RF group; and 96% and 88%, respectively, in the PEI group. Despite the tendency favoring RF ablation, the observed difference did not reach statistical significance (hazard ratio, 0.20; 95% confidence interval, 0.02–1.69; $P = 0.138$). However, 1- and 2-year recurrence-free survival rates were clearly higher in RF-treated patients than in PEI-treated patients (86% and 64%, respectively, in the RF ablation group versus 77% and 43%, respectively, in the PEI group; hazard ratio, 0.48; 95% confidence interval, 0.27–0.85; $P = 0.012$). RF treatment was confirmed as an independent prognostic factor for local recurrence-free survival by multivariate analysis.

This trial suggested that RF ablation can achieve higher recurrence-free survival rates than PEI, thereby confirming findings in two previous comparative studies, in which higher complete tumor response rates were observed in tumors treated with RF ablation with respect to those submitted to PEI [47,48]. However, likely because of the short follow-up period and the limited sample size, no difference with respect to overall survival was found. Two studies reported the long-term survival outcomes of RF ablation-treated patients (Table 3) [49,50]. In the first paper, 82 patients with small ($\leq$3.5 cm) HCC lesions were assessed in a retrospective analysis. The reported 1-, 3-, and 5-year survival rates were 89%, 62%, and 33%, respectively [49]. In the second study, 206 patients with early-stage HCC who were not candidates for resection or transplantation were enrolled in a prospective, intention-to-treat clinical trial [50]. RF ablation was considered as the first-line nonsurgical treatment, and was actually performed in 187 (91%) of 206 patients. Nineteen (9%) of 206 patients had to be excluded from RF treatment because of the unfavorable location of the tumor. Patients who were not suitable for RF ablation were treated with either PEI or segmental transcatheter arterial chemoembolization. The overall survival rates in the intention-to-treat analysis including all the 206 patients (67% at 3 years and 41% at 5 years) were not significantly different from those achieved in the 187 compliant patients who received RF ablation (71% at 3 years and 48% at 5 years; $P = 0.5094$). In patients who underwent RF ablation, survival depended on the severity of the underlying cirrhosis and the tumor multiplicity. Patients in Child class A had 3- and 5-year survival rates of 76% and 51%, respectively. This survival rate was significantly higher than that obtained in Child class B patients (46% at 3 years and 31% at 5 years; $P = 0.0006$) (Table 3). A subgroup of 116 patients in Child class A who had a solitary HCC showed 3- and 5-year survival rates of 89% and 61%, respectively.

Table 3
Studies reporting long-term survival outcomes of patients with early-stage hepatocellular carcinoma who underwent percutaneous thermal ablation

| Treatment | No. patients | Survival rates (%) 1-yr | 3-yr | 5-yr |
|---|---|---|---|---|
| Radiofrequency ablation | | | | |
| Buscarini et al, 2001 [49] | | | | |
| Child A-B, 1-3 HCCs <3.5 cm | 82 | 89 | 62 | 33 |
| Lencioni et al, 2005 [50] | | | | |
| Child A, 1 HCC <5 cm or 3 <3 cm | 144 | 100 | 76 | 51 |
| Child B, 1 HCC <5 cm or 3 <3 cm | 43 | 89 | 46 | 31 |
| Microwave ablation | | | | |
| Lu et al, 2001 [57] | 50 | 96 | 73 | NA |
| Shiina et al, 2002 [58] | 122 | 90 | 68 | NA |
| Dong et al, 2003 [59] | 234 | 93 | 73 | 57 |
| Laser ablation | | | | |
| Pacella et al, 2001 [65] | | | | |
| Child A-B, 1 HCC <4 cm or 3 <3 cm | 74 | 99 | 68 | 15 |

*Abbreviations:* NA, not available; HCC, hepatocellular carcinoma.

RF ablation is associated with acceptable morbidity. In a multicenter survey in which 2320 patients with 3554 hepatic lesions were included, six deaths (mortality rate, 0.3%) were noted, including two caused by multiorgan failure following intestinal perforation; one case each of septic shock following *Staphylococcus aureus*-caused peritonitis, massive hemorrhage following tumor rupture, liver failure following stenosis of right bile duct; and one case of sudden death of unknown cause 3 days after the procedure [51]. Fifty (2.2%) patients had additional major complications. Tumor seeding, in particular, occurred in 8 (0.5%) of 1610 HCC patients. Lesions with subcapsular location and an invasive tumoral pattern, as shown by a poor differentiation degree, seem to be at higher risk for such a complication [52]. RF ablation of superficial lesions that are adjacent to any part of the gastrointestinal tract was shown to be also at risk of thermal injury of the gastric or bowel wall [53]. Treatment of lesions adjacent to the gallbladder or to the hepatic hilum may injury the biliary tract. In experienced hands, RF ablation of tumors located in the vicinity of the gallbladder was shown to be feasible, although associated in most cases with self-limited iatrogenic cholecystitis [54].

*Microwave ablation*

Microwave ablation is the term used for all electromagnetic methods of inducing tumor destruction by using devices with frequencies greater than or equal to 900 kHz [40]. The passage of microwaves into cells or other materials containing water results in the rotation of individual molecules. This rapid molecular rotation generates and uniformly distributes heat, which is instantaneous and continuous until the radiation is stopped. Microwave irradiation creates an ablation area around the needle in a column or round shape, depending on the type of needle used and the generating power [55,56]. Three to four insertions, either simultaneously or at short intevals, may be needed to ablate tumors up to 4 cm in diameter [57].

In three uncontrolled studies of HCC patients who received microwave ablation, the 3-year survival ranged 68% to 73% (Table 3) [57–59]. One study compared microwave ablation and PEI in a retrospective evaluation of 90 patients with small HCC [60]. The overall 5-year survival rates for patients with well-differentiated HCC, treated with microwave ablation and PEI, were not significantly different. However, among the patients with moderately or poorly differentiated HCC, overall survival with microwave ablation was significantly better than with PEI ($P = 0.03$). The authors concluded that microwave ablation may be superior to PEI for the local control of moderately or poorly differentiated small HCC.

Only one randomized trial compared the effectiveness of microwave ablation with that of RF ablation [61]. Seventy-two patients with 94 HCC nodules were randomly assigned to RF ablation and microwave ablation groups. The number of treatment sessions per nodule was significantly lower in the RF ablation group than in the percutaneous microwave ablation group (1.1 versus

2.4; $P < 0.001$). Complete therapeutic effect was achieved in 46 (96%) of 48 nodules treated with RF ablation and in 41 (89%) of 46 nodules treated with percutaneous microwave ablation ($P = 0.26$). Major complications occurred in one patient treated with RF ablation and in four patients treated with percutaneous microwave ablation ($P = 0.36$). During follow-up (range, 6–27 months), residual foci of untreated disease were seen in 4 of 48 nodules treated with RF ablation and in 8 of 46 nodules treated with microwave ablation ($P = 0.20$). Unfortunately, in this study the data were analyzed with respect to lesions and not to patients. Although no statistically significant differences were observed with respect to the efficacy of the two procedures, a tendency favoring RF ablation was recognized with respect to local recurrences and complications rates [45].

### *Laser ablation*

The term laser ablation should be used for ablation with light energy applied via fibers directly inserted into the tissue. A great variety in laser sources and wavelength are available. In addition, different types of laser fibers, modified tips, and single or multiple laser applicators can be used. The laser beam consists of a coherent, monochromatic, and highly collimated beam of light. Focusing such light energy onto the liver tumor results in heat production and coagulation necrosis. From a single, bare 400-μm laser fiber, a spherical volume of coagulative necrosis up to 2 cm in diameter can be produced. Use of a higher power results in charring and vaporization around the fiber tip. Two methods have been developed for producing larger volumes of necrosis. The first consists of firing multiple bare fibers arrayed at 2-cm spacing throughout a target lesion [62], while the second uses cooled-tip diffuser fibers that can deposit up to 30 W over a large surface area, thus diminishing local overheating [63].

Most studies on laser ablation involve patients with liver metastases. To date, there are few data on the clinical efficacy of laser ablation for HCC [64,65]. In one uncontrolled study, 74 patients with either single HCC smaller than 4 cm or as many as three lesions smaller than 3 cm each were assessed. Overall survival rates were 99%, 68%, and 15% at 1, 3, and 5 years, respectively [65]. No randomized trials to compare laser ablation with any other treatment are available. The major limitation of current laser technology appears to be the small volume of ablation that can be created with a single-probe insertion. Insertion of multiple fibers is technically cumbersome, and may not be feasible in lesions that are not conveniently located.

## Open questions

Despite the many published reports, several questions concerning the clinical efficacy of local ablative therapies in the treatment of HCC are still unanswered. A number of studies have provided indirect evidence that percutaneous ablation substantially improves the natural history of patients with early-stage HCC. However, there are no data showing a clear survival benefit of newer thermal ablation techniques over the well-established PEI. Some authors have claimed that percutaneous techniques may be a safe and effective bridge to liver transplantation [66–68]. However, randomized studies are needed to determine advantages and disadvantages of local ablative treatments with respect to transcatheter arterial chemoembolization before these procedures come into general use for HCC patients in the waiting list [69]. Recent studies have reported encouraging initial results in the treatment of large HCC lesions with a combination of RF ablation and balloon catether occlusion of the tumor arterial supply or prior transcathater arterial chemobolization [70–73]. However, there are no reports showing that RF ablation in combination with intraarterial procedures improves survival in this patient population. Further randomized clinical trials are warranted to clarify these unsolved issues. Conduction and publication of such trials should be performed according to established guidelines, and sufficient follow-up should be assured [45].

## Summary

HCC is one of the most common malignancies worldwide. Only a minority of the patients can be treated by surgical resection or liver transplantation. Several minimally invasive percutaneous techniques have been developed to treat nonsurgical patients with early-stage tumors. PEI is the seminal technique for local tumor treatment, and may achieve a 5-year survival rate of 50% in selected Child A patients. RF ablation constitutes the most assessed alternative technique. On the basis of the identified evidence, RF ablation seems to reach higher recurrence-free survival rates compared with PEI. Further randomized trials are needed to establish the clinical efficacy of RF ablation with respect to other percutaneous treatments and to devise an unbiased therapeutic strategy.

## References

[1] Bruix J, Llovet JM. Prognostic prediction and treatment strategy in hepatocellular carcinoma. Hepatology 2002;35:519–24.
[2] Llovet JM, Burroughs A, Bruix J. Hepatocellular carcinoma. Lancet 2003;362:1907–17.
[3] Bruix J, Sherman M, Llovet JM, et al, EASL Panel of Experts on HCC. Clinical management of hepatocellular carcinoma. Conclusions of the Barcelona—2000 EASL conference. European Association for the Study of the Liver. J Hepatol 2001;35:421–30.
[4] Lencioni R, Cioni D, Crocetti L, et al. Percutaneous ablation of hepatocellular carcinoma: state-of-the-art. Liver Transplant 2004;10:S91–7.
[5] Dixon AK. Evidence-based diagnostic radiology. Lancet 1997;350:509–12.
[6] The Evidence-Based Radiology Working Group. Evidence-based radiology: a new approach to the practice of radiology. Radiology 2001;220:566–75.
[7] Livraghi T, Salmi A, Bolondi L, et al. Small hepatocellular carcinoma: percutaneous alcohol injection – results in 23 patients. Radiology 1988;168:313–7.

[8] Shiina S, Tagawa K, Unuma T, et al. Percutaneous ethanol injection therapy for the treatment of hepatocellular carcinoma. AJR Am J Roentgenol 1990;154:947–51.

[9] Lencioni R, Caramella D, Bartolozzi C. Response of hepatocellular carcinoma to percutaneous ethanol injection: CT and MR evaluation. J Comput Assist Tomogr 1993;17:723–9.

[10] Shiina S, Tagawa K, Unuma T, et al. Percutaneous ethanol injection therapy for hepatocellular carcinoma: a histopathologic study. Cancer 1991;68:1524–30.

[11] Shiina S, Tagawa K, Niwa Y, et al. Percutaneous ethanol injection therapy for hepatocellular carcinoma: results in 146 patients. AJR Am J Roentgenol 1993;160:1023–8.

[12] Lencioni R, Bartolozzi C, Caramella D, et al. Treatment of small hepatocellular carcinoma with percutaneous ethanol injection. Analysis of prognostic factors in 105 Western patients. Cancer 1995;76:1737–46.

[13] Livraghi T, Giorgio A, Marin G, et al. Hepatocellular carcinoma and cirrhosis in 746 patients: long-term results of percutaneous ethanol injection. Radiology 1995;197:101–8.

[14] Ryu M, Shimamura Y, Kinoshita T, et al. Therapeutic results of resection, transcatheter arterial embolization and percutaneous transhepatic ethanol injection in 3225 patients with hepatocellular carcinoma: a retrospective multicenter study. Jpn J Clin Oncol 1997;27:251–7.

[15] Lencioni R, Pinto F, Armillotta N, et al. Long-term results of percutaneous ethanol injection therapy for hepatocellular carcinoma in cirrhosis: a European experience. Eur Radiol 1997;7: 514–9.

[16] Pompili M, Rapaccini GL, Covino M, et al. Prognostic factors for survival in patients with compensated cirrhosis and small hepatocellular carcinoma after percutaneous ethanol injection therapy. Cancer 2001;92:126–35.

[17] Teratani T, Ishikawa T, Shiratori Y, et al. Hepatocellular carcinoma in elderly patients: beneficial therapeutic efficacy using percutaneous ethanol injection therapy. Cancer 2002; 95:816–23.

[18] The Liver Cancer Study Group of Japan. Primary liver cancer in Japan. Ann Surg 1990;221: 277–87.

[19] Livraghi T, Bolondi L, Buscarini L, et al. No treatment, resection and ethanol injection in hepatocellular carcinoma: a retrospective analysis of survival in 391 patients with cirrhosis. Italian Cooperative HCC Study Group. J Hepatol 1995;22:522–6.

[20] Castells A, Bruix J, Bru C, et al. Treatment of small hepatocellular carcinoma in cirrhotic patients: a cohort study comparing surgical resection and percutaneous ethanol injection. Hepatology 1993;18:1121–6.

[21] Yamamoto J, Okada S, Shimada K, et al. Treatment strategy for small hepatocellular carcinoma: comparison of long-term results after percutaneous ethanol injection therapy and surgical resection. Hepatology 2001;34:707–13.

[22] Daniele B, De Sio I, Izzo F, et al, CLIP Investigators. Hepatic resection and percutaneous ethanol injection as treatments of small hepatocellular carcinoma: a Cancer of the Liver Italian Program (CLIP 08) retrospective case–control study. J Clin Gastroenterol 2003;36:63–7.

[23] Di Stasi M, Buscarini L, Livraghi T, et al. Percutaneous ethanol injection in the treatment of hepatocellular carcinoma. A multicenter survey of evaluation practices and complication rates. Scand J Gastroenterol 1997;32:1168–73.

[24] Khan KN, Yatsuhashi H, Yamasaki K, et al. Prospective analysis of risk factors for early intrahepatic recurrence of hepatocellular carcinoma following ethanol injection. J Hepatol 2000;32:269–78.

[25] Koda M, Murawaki Y, Mitsuda A, et al. Predictive factors for intrahepatic recurrence after percutaneous ethanol injection therapy for small hepatocellular carcinoma. Cancer 2000;88: 529–37.

[26] Okusaka T, Okada S, Ueno H, et al. Satellite lesions in patients with small hepatocellular carcinoma with reference to clinicopathologic features. Cancer 2002;95:1931–7.

[27] Livraghi T, Benedini V, Lazzaroni S, et al. Long-term results of single-session percutaneous ethanol injection in patients with large hepatocellular carcinoma. Cancer 1998;83:48–57.

[28] Llovet JM, Bustamante J, Castells A, et al. Natural history of untreated nonsurgical

hepatocellular carcinoma: rationale for the design and evaluation of therapeutic trials. Hepatology 1999;29:62–7.

[29] Ohnishi K, Yoshioka H, Ito S, et al. Treatment of nodular hepatocellular carcinoma larger than 3 cm with ultrasound-guided percutaneous acetic acid injection. Hepatology 1996;24:1379–85.

[30] Honda N, Guo Q, Uchida H, et al. Percutaneous hot saline injection therapy for hepatic tumors: an alternative to percutaneous ethanol injection therapy. Radiology 1994;190:53–7.

[31] Ohnishi K, Yoshioka H, Ito S, et al. Prospective randomized controlled trial comparing percutaneous acetic acid injection and percutaneous ethanol injection for small hepatocellular carcinoma. Hepatology 1998;27:67–72.

[32] Huo TI, Huang YH, Wu JC, et al. Comparison of percutaneous acetic acid injection and percutaneous ethanol injection for hepatocellular carcinoma in cirrhotic patients: a prospective study. Scand J Gastroenterol 2003;38:770–8.

[33] Yoon HK, Song HY, Sung KB, et al. Percutaneous hot saline injection therapy: effectiveness in large hepatocellular carcinoma. J Vasc Interv Radiol 1999;10:477–82.

[34] Goldberg SN, Gazelle GS, Mueller PR. Thermal ablation therapy for focal malignancies: a unfied approach to underlyng principles, techniques, and diagnostic imaging guidance. AJR Am J Roentgenol 2000;174:323–31.

[35] Goldberg SN, Gazelle GS, Halpern EF, et al. Radiofrequency tissue ablation: importance of local temperature along the electrode tip exposure in determining lesion size and shape. Acad Radiol 1996;3:212–8.

[36] Lencioni R, Goletti O, Armillotta N, et al. Radio-frequency thermal ablation of liver metastases with a cooled-tip electrode needle: results of a pilot clinical trial. Eur Radiol 1998; 8:1205–11.

[37] Rossi S, Buscarini E, Garbagnati F, et al. Percutaneous treatment of small hepatic tumors by an expandable RF needle electrode. AJR Am J Roentgenol 1998;170:1015–22.

[38] Goldberg SN, Solbiati L, Hahn PF, et al. Large volume tissue ablation with radiofrequency by using a clustered, internally cooled electrode technique: laboratory and clinical experience in liver metastases. Radiology 1998;209:371–9.

[39] Lencioni R, Cioni D, Bartolozzi C. Percutaneous radiofrequency thermal ablation of liver malignancies: techniques, indications, imaging findings, and clinical results. Abdom Imaging 2001;26:345–60.

[40] Goldberg SN, Charboneau JW, Dodd 3rd GD, et al, International Working Group on Image-Guided Tumor Ablation. Image-guided tumor ablation: proposal for standardization of terms and reporting criteria. Radiology 2003;228:335–45.

[41] Lencioni R, Crocetti L, Cioni D, et al. Percutaneous radiofrequency ablation of hepatic colorectal metastases. Technique, indications, results, and new promises. Invest Radiol 2004; 39:689–97.

[42] Curley SA, Izzo F, Delrio P, et al. Radiofrequency ablation of unresectable primary and metastatic malignancies: results in 123 patients. Ann Surg 1999;230:1–8.

[43] Jiao LR, Hansen PD, Havlik R, et al. Clinical short-term results of radiofrequency ablation in primary and secondary liver tumors. Am J Surg 1999;177:303–6.

[44] Wood TF, Rose DM, Chung M, et al. Radiofrequency ablation of 231 unresectable hepatic tumors: indications, limitations, and complications. Ann Surg Oncol 2000;7:593–600.

[45] Galandi D, Antes G. Radiofrequency thermal ablation versus other interventions for hepatocellular carcinoma (Cochrane Review). In: The Cochrane Library, issue 2. Chichester: John Wiley & Sons, Ltd; 2004.

[46] Lencioni R, Allgaier HP, Cioni D, et al. Small hepatocellular carcinoma in cirrhosis: randomized comparison of radiofrequency thermal ablation versus percutaneous ethanol injection. Radiology 2003;228:235–40.

[47] Livraghi T, Goldberg SN, Lazzaroni S, et al. Small hepatocellular carcinoma: treatment with radio-frequency ablation versus ethanol injection. Radiology 1999;210:655–61.

[48] Ikeda M, Okada S, Ueno H, et al. Radiofrequency ablation and percutaneous ethanol injection in patients with small hepatocellular carcinoma: a comparative study. Jpn J Clin Oncol 2001; 31:322–6.

[49] Buscarini L, Buscarini E, Di Stasi M, et al. Percutaneous radiofrequency ablation of small hepatocellular carcinoma: long-term results. Eur Radiol 2001;11:914–21.
[50] Lencioni R, Cioni D, Crocetti L, et al. Early-stage hepatocellular carcinoma in cirrhosis: long-term results of percutaneous image-guided radiofrequency ablation. Radiology 2005 [In press].
[51] Livraghi T, Solbiati L, Meloni MF, et al. Treatment of focal liver tumors with percutaneous radio-frequency ablation: complications encountered in a multicenter study. Radiology 2003; 226:441–51.
[52] Llovet JM, Vilana R, Bru C, et al, Barcelona Clinic Liver Cancer (BCLC) Group. Increased risk of tumor seeding after percutaneous radiofrequency ablation for single hepatocellular carcinoma. Hepatology 2001;33:1124–9.
[53] Rhim H, Dodd 3rd GD, Chintapalli KN, et al. Radiofrequency thermal ablation of abdominal tumors: lessons learned from complications. Radiographics 2004;24:41–52.
[54] Chopra S, Dodd 3rd GD, Chanin MP, et al. Radiofrequency ablation of hepatic tumors adjacent to the gallbladder: feasibility and safety. AJR Am J Roentgenol 2003;180:697–701.
[55] Seki T, Wakabayashi M, Nakagawa T, et al. Ultrasonically guided percutaneous microwave coagulation therapy for small hepatocellular carcinoma. Cancer 1994;74:817–25.
[56] Sato M, Watanabe Y, Ueda S, et al. Microwave coagulation therapy for hepatocellular carcinoma. Gastroenterology 1996;110:1507–14.
[57] Lu MD, Chen JW, Xie XY, et al. Hepatocellular carcinoma: US-guided percutaneous microwave coagulation therapy. Radiology 2001;221:167–72.
[58] Shiina S, Teratani T, Obi S, et al. Nonsurgical treatment of hepatocellular carcinoma: from percutaneous ethanol injection therapy and percutaneous microwave coagulation therapy to radiofrequency ablation. Oncology 2002;62(Suppl 1):64–8.
[59] Dong B, Liang P, Yu X, et al. Percutaneous sonographically guided microwave coagulation therapy for hepatocellular carcinoma: results in 234 patients. AJR Am J Roentgenol 2003;180: 1547–55.
[60] Seki T, Wakabayashi M, Nakagawa T, et al. Percutaneous microwave coagulation therapy for patients with small hepatocellular carcinoma: comparison with percutaneous ethanol injection therapy. Cancer 1999;85:1694–702.
[61] Shibata T, Iimuro Y, Yamamoto Y, et al. Small hepatocellular carcinoma: comparison of radio-frequency ablation and percutaneous microwave coagulation therapy. Radiology 2002; 223:331–7.
[62] Steger AC, Lees WR, Walmsley K, et al. Interstitial laser hyperthermia: a new approach to local destruction of tumours. BMJ 1989;299:362–5.
[63] Vogl TJ, Muller PK, Hammerstingl R, et al. Malignant liver tumors treated with MR imaging-guided laser-induced thermotherapy: technique and prospective results. Radiology 1995;196:257–65.
[64] Christophi C, Muralidharan V. Treatment of hepatocellular carcinoma by percutaneous laser hyperthermia. J Gastroenterol Hepatol 2001;16:548–52.
[65] Pacella CM, Bizzarri G, Magnolfi F, et al. Laser thermal ablation in the treatment of small hepatocellular carcinoma: results in 74 patients. Radiology 2001;221:712–20.
[66] Kato T, Tamura S, Tekin A, et al. Use of microwave coagulation therapy in liver transplant candidates with hepatocellular carcinoma: a preliminary report. Transplant Proc 2001;33:1469.
[67] Fontana RJ, Hamidullah H, Nghiem H, et al. Percutaneous radiofrequency thermal ablation of hepatocellular carcinoma: a safe and effective bridge to liver transplantation. Liver Transplant 2002;8:1165–74.
[68] Wong LL, Tanaka K, Lau L, et al. Pre-transplant treatment of hepatocellular carcinoma: assessment of tumor necrosis in explanted livers. Clin Transplant 2004;18:227–34.
[69] Graziadei IW, Sandmueller H, Waldenberger P, et al. Chemoembolization followed by liver transplantation for hepatocellular carcinoma impedes tumor progression while on the waiting list and leads to excellent outcome. Liver Transplant 2003;9:557–63.
[70] Rossi S, Garbagnati F, Lencioni R, et al. Percutaneous radio-frequency thermal ablation of

nonresectable hepatocellular carcinoma after occlusion of tumor blood supply. Radiology 2000;217:119–26.

[71] Yamasaki T, Kurokawa F, Shirahashi H, et al. Percutaneous radiofrequency ablation therapy for patients with hepatocellular carcinoma during occlusion of hepatic blood flow. Comparison with standard percutaneous radiofrequency ablation therapy. Cancer 2002;95:2353–60.

[72] Yamakado K, Nakatsuka A, Ohmori S, et al. Radiofrequency ablation combined with chemoembolization in hepatocellular carcinoma: treatment response based on tumor size and morphology. J Vasc Interv Radiol 2002;13:1225–32.

[73] Kitamoto M, Imagawa M, Yamada H, et al. Radiofrequency ablation in the treatment of small hepatocellular carcinomas: comparison of the radiofrequency effect with and without chemoembolization. AJR Am J Roentgenol 2003;181:997–1003.

ELSEVIER
SAUNDERS

Clin Liver Dis 9 (2005) 315–328

CLINICS IN
LIVER DISEASE

# Liver Transplantation for Hepatocellular Carcinoma: Is Expansion of Criteria Justified?

Sasan Roayaie, MD[a], Josep M. Llovet, MD[a,b,*]

[a]*Division of Liver Diseases and Recanati/Miller Transplantation Institute, Mount Sinai School of Medicine, Madison Avenue 1425, 11F-70, Box 1123, New York, NY 10029, USA*
[b]*BCLC Group, Liver Unit, Digestive Disease Institute, IDIBAPS, Hospital Clínic, University of Barcelona, Catalonia, Spain*

Hepatocellular carcinoma (HCC) is a major health problem worldwide, involving more than a half million new cases yearly, with an age-adjusted incidence of 5.5 to 14.9 per $10^5$ population [1]. In some areas of Asia and the Middle East, HCC ranks as the first cause of death due to cancer. The incidence of HCC is increasing in Europe and the United States [2], and it is currently the leading cause of death among cirrhotic patients [3]. It is estimated that by the year 2010, the number of patients with HCC awaiting liver transplant in the United States will outnumber the supply of cadaver organs.

## Overview of treatments for hepatocellular carcinoma

In Western countries, surveillance programs have lead to an increase in the applicability of radical therapies, with 30% to 40% of the patients being eligible for such treatments in referral centers [4]. There is no firm evidence to establish the optimal first-line treatment for a small single HCC in patients with well-preserved liver function [5]. This is due to the fact that there are no randomized controlled trials comparing any of the three major radical therapies: resection,

Josep M. Llovet is supported by a grant from AGAUR (2004BE00226, Generalitat de Catalunya, Spain), Instituto de Salud Carlos III (Fondo de Investigaciones Sanitarias 2002-2005, PI02/0596) and Programa "Ramon y Cajal" (IDIBAPS, Ministerio de Ciencia y Tecnologia, Spain).

* Corresponding author. Division of Liver Diseases and Recanati/Miller Transplantation Institute, Mount Sinai School of Medicine, 19 East 98th St, Suite 6F, Box 1104, New York, NY 10029.
*E-mail address:* Josep.Llovet@mssm.edu (J.M. Llovet).

1089-3261/05/$ – see front matter 
doi:10.1016/j.cld.2004.12.007

liver transplantation (LT), and percutaneous treatments. These studies are not feasible in the West due to the need for a large sample size and the resources required. Recent attempts to compare resection versus percutaneous treatments have failed both in Italy and Japan, although at least one new study is being conducted in Asia. Evidence of relative benefit is derived from numerous non-randomized cohort studies. At present, resection and transplantation achieve the best outcomes in well-selected candidates (5-year survival of 60–70%), and compete as the first option from an intention-to-treat perspective [6,7]. LT can be applied to around 10% to 20% of patients seen at referral centers, but to less than 5% if the whole HCC population is considered. If surgery is precluded, local, nonsurgical therapies are applied. Percutaneous treatments provide good results (5-year survival of 40–50%), but are unable to achieve response rates and outcomes comparable to surgical treatments, even when applied as the first option [8,9]. The remaining treatments have been assessed in the setting of around 70 randomized controlled trials conducted during the last 25 years [10]. In these studies only chemoembolization has been shown to improve survival in around 10% of the whole HCC population [11]. Internal radiation and intraarterial chemotherapy provide promising results, but are without any proven impact on survival. Tamoxifen does not provide survival advantages. Clinical data assessing new generations of drugs such as cytostatic agents, immunomodulators, or gene therapies is still scarce.

## Liver transplantation for hepatocellular carcinoma: Historic perspective

The clinical impact of LT has changed the treatment strategy for HCC, particularly in the West. In well-selected candidates, this treatment may potentially cure the tumor and the underlying cirrhosis at the same time. However, the role of LT in the management of HCC has evolved throughout three different periods.

During the 1980s, the high recurrence rate (32–54%) and poor outcomes (5-year survival $<40\%$) obtained from transplant registries were related to the acceptance of exceedingly advanced tumors with adverse prognostic factors such as macroscopic vascular invasion, lymph node involvement, and extra-hepatic spread at the time of the procedure [12–15] (Table 1). These devastating figures questioned the indication of LT for HCC in some programs. The initial experiences, however, served to demonstrate the feasibility of the operation and to establish the criteria that avoided a very aggressive and expensive treatment in patients with no option for long-term survival. The second era of LT for HCC started during the early 1990s. The analysis of the previous experience suggested that patients with minute or incidental asymptomatic tumors discovered at the time of transplantation had the same outcome as patients with nonmalignant disease [16]. Some pioneering groups selecting the "optimal candidates"—patients with single HCC $\leq 5$ cm or up to three nodules $\leq 3$ cm—reported a 70% 5-year survival with a recurrence rate below 15% [17–20]

Table 1
First series of liver transplantation for HCC

| Authors | N | Tumor stage | Recurrence | Survival 3 yr | Survival 5 yr |
|---|---|---|---|---|---|
| Ringe et al., 1991 [12] | 61 | 80% > 5 cm | — | 15% | 15% |
| Iwatsuki et al., 1991 [13] | 105 | 35% portal invasion<br>75% multinodular | 43% | 39% | 36% |
| Bismuth et al., 1993 [14] | 60 | 50% symptomatic<br>50% > 3 nodules<br>17% Portal invasion | 54% | 49% | — |
| Moreno et al., 1995 [15] | 38 | 25% portal invasion<br>60% T4. | 32% | 67% | 48% |

*Abbreviation:* HCC, hepatocellular carcinoma.

(Table 2). This was first proposed by Bismuth et al [14], refined later by Mazzaferro et al [7], and ultimately confirmed by several other groups [17,19]. During this period, LT was considered in most centers as the first-line option for early HCC. Years later, the United Network for Organ Sharing (UNOS) adapted this definition to provide priority to HCC patients enlisted for LT. More recently, the federal government of the United States approved full financial coverage by Medicare for patients being transplanted for HCC.

When dissecting all these studies it became clear that they shared not only a strict selection criteria, but also a short waiting time of less than 6 months. A thorough analysis of the outcomes reported led to the appreciation that only vascular invasion, or its surrogates markers—such as poor tumor differentiation—were able to alter the prognosis of well-selected candidates by causing recurrence in a minority of patients [19,21–25]. Other tumor-related prognostic factors were recognized only when including patients at more advanced stages [13,14] (Table 3). In addition, the tumor node metastases (TNM) classification was questioned as an efficient tool for HCC staging before LT, and became a marginal staging system in clinical practice [17]. At this point, the ideal candidates for LT were already recognized, and a common agreement was that patients should only be listed for LT when the probability of living 5 years after the procedure exceeded 50% [26].

Table 2
Outcomes of patients with early HCC treated by liver transplantation: Restrictive selection criteria

| Author (journal, year) | N | Recurrence | Survival 1 yr | Survival 5 yr |
|---|---|---|---|---|
| Mazzaferro et al., N Engl J Med 1996 [7] | 48 | 8% | 84% | 74%[a] |
| Bismuth et al., Semin Liver Dis 1999 [18] | 45 | 11% | 82% | 74% |
| Llovet et al., Hepatology 1999 [6] | 79 | 4% | 86% | 75% |
| Intention-to-treat analysis | 87 | | 84% | 69% |
| Jonas et al., Hepatology 2001 [19] | 120 | 16% | 90% | 71% |

*Abbreviation:* HCC, hepatocellular carcinoma.
[a] 4–yr survival.

Table 3
Predictors of recurrence of HCC after CLT: Multivariate analysis

| Study | n | Predictors of recurrence |
|---|---|---|
| Iwatsuki, 1991 [13] | 105 | Bilobar tumor, lymph node metastases<br>Vascular invasion[a], positive margins |
| Bismuth, 1993 [14][b] | 60 | Size, number of tumors, portal thrombus |
| Roayaie, 2000 [21] | 119 | Size, vascular invasion[a] |
| Jonas, 2001 [19] | 120 | Vascular invasion[a], tumor grade |
| Hemming, 2002 [23] | 112 | Vascular invasion[a] |
| Llovet, 2003 [22] | 172 | Vascular invasion[a] |
| Shetty, 2004[b] [24] | 109 | Macrovascular invasion, AFP |
| Todo, 2004 [25] | 316 | Size, AFP, bilobar disease, vascular invasion[a] |

*Abbreviations:* AFP, α-fentoprotein; CLT, cadaveric liver transplantation.
[a] Includes micro- and macrovascular invasion.
[b] Only univariate analysis available.

At present, we face a new situation, with two opposing driving forces in the field. First, there was the evidence that the shortage of donors has led to extremely long waiting times in almost all countries, resulting in a distortion of reported outcomes when analyzed according to intention to treat [6,27,28]. Second, an increasing number of studies propose that the expansion of the conventional criteria may not adversely impact survival [29–32]. To our knowledge, no single approach has attempted to analyze both phenomena together, and thus we are going to dissect them separately.

## Dropout rate and survival according to intention to treat

The Barcelona (BCLC) group reported the impact of dropout on overall survival in HCC patients enlisted for LT [6], and these results have been confirmed by other groups [27,28]. In our study, dropout rates above 20% in waiting times exceeding 6 months lead to alarming survival figures according to intention to treat (around 60% at 2 years). Today, leading programs in the United States and Europe face a waiting time of over 12 months, and UNOS data indicate that the number of patients excluded while waiting almost equals the number that are effectively transplanted. The dropout rate may account for 20% to 30% of cases [27], and is a major clinical problem for most Transplant Programs. This event is also common, but less frequent, in patients listed without HCC, and has brought into question the system for allocation of livers. In the United States, UNOS adopted the Model for End-Stage Liver Disease system to allocate organs according to a composite score that includes bilirubin, prothrombin activity, and creatinine levels for noncancer patients, and a variable score between 24 to 29 points for HCC patients [33]. This score has been recently modified to ascribe 24 points to HCC patients with tumors $\geq 2$ cm in diameter. The fact that the priority policy adopted by the UNOS has been evolving during the last years (reviewed elsewhere [34]) makes it difficult to translate the American experience to centers outside the Untied States. We have recently analyzed the predictors of dropout in a cohort of 201 HCC patients enlisted for LT and identified baseline α-fetoprotein levels >200 ng/mL, tumors >3 cm in diameter, tumor doubling time <6 months, and treatment failure as independent predictors of dropout [22]. These factors might provide the basis of a rational priority policy.

Several strategies have been proposed to ameliorate the impact of tumor progression while waiting for a donor. The adjuvant therapies—percutaneous ablation, chemoembolization, or even chemotherapy—applied while waiting for LT, have been assessed in the setting of observational studies [17,25,35]. At present, there is no evidence of survival benefit for these procedures, and thus randomized studies are needed to assess whether neo-adjuvant therapies might decrease the dropout rate or prevent recurrences after transplantation. Only cost-effectiveness analysis using the Markov model suggested a survival advantage of 6 months for adjuvant therapies using resection or percutaneous treatment in comparison to conservative treatments [36]. Marginal livers, domino, and split transplantation represent alternatives that only solve a minor proportion of cases.

## Assessment of extended indications

The standard selection criteria for cadaveric LT (CLT) rely upon a strict size limitation. These criteria have been recently questioned, and some groups are proposing extended indications for HCC [29–32]. To further analyze the rationale of these proposals, at least three considerations should be taken into account. First, it is important to define whether the proposed expanded criteria are based on preoperative radiologic imaging and staging at the time of presentation for LT, or whether they are based upon pathologic staging using the explanted liver. Second, the reported outcomes should take into account the potential increased dropout rates that will occur as a result of selecting patients at a more advanced stage of the disease. In fact, one of the major concerns is that relaxation of the current guidelines would further lengthen time spent on the waiting list, which in turn, may increase the withdrawal rates and worsen intention-to-treat outcomes. Finally, it is important analyze the results obtained with CLT separately from living donor LT (LDLT), because it is not completely proven that both procedures provide equivalent outcomes.

### *Disease extension: Radiology versus pathology*

Diagnosis and staging of HCC are crucial to establish the indications for LT. An accurate pretreatment staging is critical to detect minute intrahepatic metastases, the equivalent to minimal residual disease in other neoplasms. The accuracy of ultrasound for HCC detection is high, and comparable to helical CT scan or magnetic resonance imaging (MRI). It is more difficult to determine the extension of the disease beyond the primary lesion. Ultrasound is unable to

Table 4
Comparison between radiological and pathological HCC staging of the explanted livers

| Authors | N | Selection criteria | Accurate disease extension |
|---|---|---|---|
| Rizzi, Gastroenterology 1994 [39] | 30 | Multinodular HCC | 74% |
| Mazzaferro, N Engl J Med 1996 [7] | 45 | Single <3 cm<br>3 nodules <3 cm | 70% |
| Yao, Hepatology 2001 [30] | 64 | Single <6.5 cm<br>3 nodules <4.5 cm | 76% |
| De Carlis, J Am Coll Surg 2003 [40] | 121 | Single <3 cm<br>3 nodules <3 cm | 69% |
| Burrel, Hepatology 2003 [41] | 76 | Single <3 cm<br>3 nodules <3 cm | 76% |

*Abbreviation:* HCC, hepatocellular carcinoma.

identify small additional nodules, mostly below 1 to 2 cm [37]. Other invasive techniques have significant limitations either due to their invasiveness, such as CT during hepatic arteriography, which requires selective arteriography, or due to their low specificity, such as with lipiodol CT [37]. Today, CT scan and MRI compete as the best available technologies, with accuracies estimated around 80% [38]. However, studies investigating liver explants showed sensitivities for HCC detection with helical CT or MRI, in a per-nodule basis, ranging from 37% to 78% [17,30,39–41] (Table 4). We recently demonstrated that MRI-angiography was significantly better than triphasic helical CT in detection of HCC nodules (76% versus 61%), particularly in additional nodules between 10 to 20 mm in diameter (84% versus 47%) [41] (Table 5). Thus, even with state-

Table 5
Sensitivity of MRA and helical CT for detection of main HCC and additional nodules prior transplantation, as compared with explanted livers

| Variables | Pathology | MRA[a] | CT[b] | *P* |
|---|---|---|---|---|
| Per-nodule basis (n = 76)[a] | | | | |
| All HCC nodules | 76 | 76% | 61% | 0.001 |
| >20 mm | 25 | 100% | 100% | NS |
| 10–20 mm | 28 | 89% | 65% | 0.03 |
| <10 mm | 23 | 34% | 10% | 0.06 |
| Main nodules | 29 | 100% | 100% | NS |
| Additional nodules | 47 | 61% | 38% | 0.001 |
| >20 mm | 6 | 100% | 100% | NS |
| 10–20 mm | 19 | 84% | 47% | 0.016 |
| <10 mm | 22 | 32% | 10% | NS |

*Abbreviation:* HCC, hepatocellular carcinoma.

[a] MRA: MRI-angiography was performed in 50 cirrhotic patients. Twenty-nine patients presented 76 nodules.

[b] Helical CT: triphasic helical CT was performed in 26 of 29 HCC patients, presenting a total of 70 nodules.

*Adapted from* Burrel M, Llovet JM, Ayuso C, et al. MRI angiography is superior to helical CT for detection of HCC prior to liver transplantation: an explant correlation. Hepatology 2003;38:1034–42; with permission.

of-the-art equipment [42,43] we will always have some degree of understaging, mostly due to the failure to detect very small additional nodules < 1 cm and or microscopic vascular invasion. Therefore, the proposals for expansion of HCC listing criteria based on explant examination should take into account no imaging techniques have been shown to have the same diagnostic accuracy as pathology.

Recently, several studies have been published assessing expanded HCC indications for CLT [29–32,44] (Table 6). Two groups have proposed expanded indications based on retrospective analysis of the pathologic reports [30,31], whereas other groups assessed a prospective application of expanded criteria based on preoperative imaging techniques [29,43].

A retrospective study of 70 HCC patients from the University from California–San Francisco undergoing LT proposed a new tumor staging classification (one tumor ≤ 6.5 cm or up to three tumors ≤ 4.5 and total tumor diameter ≤ 8 cm) [30]. The overall survival of the patients meeting the new criteria (n = 60) at 1 and 5 years was 90% and 75%, significantly better than those outside the criteria. As noted by the authors and other groups, though, the proportion of patients meeting the expanded criteria was small—around 5% of all enlisted [24,31]. The major concerns of this proposal are the lack of specific data on overall survival and dropout rate on the waiting list for the patients outside the current criteria but fulfilling the expanded criteria [30]. The group of the University of Pittsburgh has also retrospectively reviewed the pathology reports of 393 patients undergoing liver transplant, and classified the subjects according to three of the different staging systems [31]. Although the reported recurrence rates were not strikingly different (3.6% versus 9% Milan versus

Table 6
Extended indications for HCC in patients undergoing cadaveric liver transplantation

| | | N | | 5-year survival | |
|---|---|---|---|---|---|
| Author, year | Design and selection criteria | All | Beyond Milan | All | Beyond Milan |
| Herrero, 2001 [29] | Prospective. Pre-LT, radiology<br>One tumor ≤ 6 cm<br>3 tumors ≤ 5 cm | 49 | 12 | 79% | N/A |
| Yao, 2001 [30] | Retrospective. Post-LT, pathology<br>One tumor ≤ 6.5 cm or<br>3 tumors ≤ 4.5 cm<br>Total tumor diameter ≤ 8.0 cm | 70 | N/A | 75% | N/A |
| Roayaie, 2002 [43] | Prospective. Pre-LT, radiology<br>Any HCC, no extrahepatic spread<br>No main portal invasion. | 80 | 80 | 25% | 25%[a]<br>43 LT:44% |
| Marsh, 2003 [31] | Retrospective. Post-LT, pathology | 393 | 145 | N/A | N/A |
| Cillo, 2004 [32] | Prospective. Pre-LT, pathology<br>Well-mod differentiated | 33 | 13 | 75% | N/A |

*Abbreviations:* HCC, hepatocellular carcinoma; LT, liver transplantation.

[a] 5-year survival according to intention to treat: 25%. 5-year survival of patients effectively transplanted: 44%.

Pittsburg criteria), no survival data of patients exceeding the conventional limits was provided.

*Expansion of criteria and dropout*

One of the major concerns of the above studies is the fact that if the tumors were listed at a more advanced stage, dropout while waiting would sharply increase. Very few studies have addressed this issue, which is crucial to understand the potential impact of using expanded pathologic criteria as a baseline decision-making criteria prior to transplantation. Recently, a prospective study from Mount Sinai reported a series of 80 patients with HCC exceeding the Milan criteria but without main portal vein invasion (although macrovascular invasion of intrahepatic portal branches was permissible) or extrahepatic spread, who were enlisted for LT [43]. Patients received preoperative chemoembolization and adjuvant treatment with systemic doxorubicin. Mean waiting time was 142 days, and 37 patients were eventually excluded due to disease progression (dropout rate: 46%). The overall 5-year intention-to-treat survival

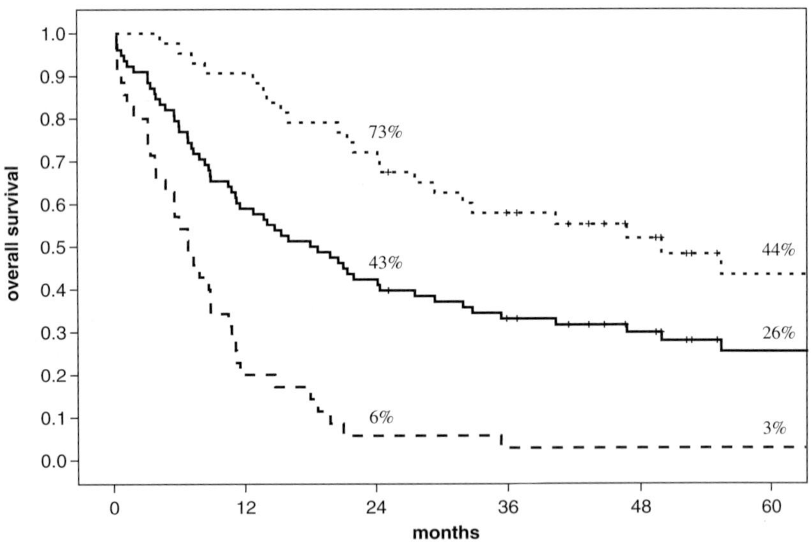


| Patients at risk | | | | | | |
|---|---|---|---|---|---|---|
| Intention to treat | 80 | 46 | 33 | 24 | 17 | 10 |
| Transplanted | 43 | 39 | 31 | 23 | 16 | 9 |
| Dropped-out | 37 | 7 | 2 | 1 | 1 | 1 |

Fig. 1. Survival of 80 patients with expanded criteria for HCC enlisted for CLT. Overall intention-to-treat survival (n = 80, 5-year survival: 25%, full line). Survival of patients effectively transplanted (n = 43, 5-year survival 44%, dotted line). Survival of patient dropping out from the waiting list due to tumor progression (n = 37, 2-year survival 5%, dashed line). (*Modified from* Roayaie S, Frischer J, Emre SH, et al. Long-term results with multimodal adjuvant therapy and liver transplantation for the treatment of hepatocellular carcinomas larger than 5 cm. Ann Surg 2002;235:533–9; with permission.)

was of 25% (Fig. 1). Among the patients effectively transplanted, 5-year survival rates above 50% were achieved in patients with tumors of 5 to 7 cm in diameter without vascular invasion. This demonstrates that the group of patients with expanded criteria is obviously heterogeneous, and that there might be room for selection refinement.

Few other prospective studies have been reported, and no compelling evidence of the benefit of expanded indications has been provided. Two studies from Europe proposed a modest expansion of the criteria either based on tumor size (single $\leq 6$ cm or up to three tumors $\leq 5$ cm) [29] or based on exclusion of patients with poor tumor differentiation, regardless of tumor size [32]. The major drawback of these studies is that only a few patients with expanded indications beyond the Milan criteria were included (12 and 13, respectively). This limitation may explain why this variable was not identified as a prognostic predictor in the multivariate analysis, despite a trend in survival analysis.

*Expanded indications according to the type of transplantation: CLT versus living donor liver transplantation*

With the limited pool of cadaveric donors, LDLT has become the most feasible alternative to cadaveric LT (CLT) for patients with end-stage liver disease or HCC. Today, more than 4000 LDLT have been performed worldwide using the right hepatic lobe. Despite this high number of procedures, the enthusiasm for LDLT is tempered by the need of a highly skilled group of senior liver surgeons, the elevated surgical-related morbidity, and the potential for donor mortality [45]. In addition, the applicability of LDLT is low, and only one fourth or less of potential recipients eventually undergo the procedure.

As stated above, the selection of candidates should rely upon preestablished preoperative staging. On the contrary, the principle of expanded criteria may apply to LDLT, considering the potential unlimited availability of a donor organ as well as the almost negligible waiting time. However, the scientific community assumed that outcomes after LDLT and CLT were comparable, and this provided the rationale to propose LDLT in patients awaiting CLT. Consequently, cost-effectiveness analyses were run with those assumptions [46]. Although there are studies reporting similar outcomes for both groups [47], others suggest that HCV disease recurrence has an earlier and more severe course in LDLT compared with CLT [48]. These data should be considered to avoid a bias in the interpretation of the results.

The majority of series reporting outcomes of LDLT in patients with HCC have a short follow-up, and thus, only early recurrences are available [25,44, 49–52] (Table 7). Following the Milan criteria the 1-year recurrence is 5% or less. Beyond these criteria the outcome is heterogeneous, ranging between 0% to 20%. As expected, unacceptable recurrence rates of 15% or above are described in patients with preoperative macroscopic vascular invasion [41–52]. The BCLC group proposed a set of criteria expecting to achieve 50% 5-year survival rates in patients with either single tumors $\leq 7$ cm, three nodules $\leq 5$ cm, five nodules

Table 7
Extended indications for HCC in patients undergoing cadaveric liver transplantation

| Author, year (n) | N | Selection criteria | Recurrence | Survival |
|---|---|---|---|---|
| Steinmuller, Transplant Proc 2002 [44] | 10 | Any HCC, vascular invasion | 20% | N/A |
| BCLC group, Liver Transpl 2003 [50] | 12 | Single <7 cm<br>3 <5 cm or 5 <3 cm | 0% | N/A |
| Kaihara, Transplantation 2003 [51] | 56 | Any HCC, no vascular invasion | | 3 year—54% |
| | | Milan criteria | 5% | |
| | | Beyond Milan criteria | 15% | |
| Gondolesi, Ann Surg 2004 [52] | 36 | Any HCC, no vascular invasion | 17% | 2 year—60% |
| | | Milan criteria (15) | | |
| | | Beyond Milan criteria (21) | | |
| Todo, Ann Surg 2004 [25] | 316 | Any HCC, no vascular invasion | | |
| | | Milan criteria (137) | 2% | 3 year—79% |
| | | Beyond Milan criteria (172) | 20% | 3 year—60% |

*Abbreviation:* HCC, hepatocellular carcinoma.

$\leq$3 cm, or downstaging to conventional criteria after any therapy lasting more than 6 months [26]. Although the results are preliminary, no recurrences have been detected with 12 cases at this point [50].

Only three series of LDLT for HCC provide survival outcomes [25,51,52]. The first study from Japan including 56 patients reported a 3-year survival rate of 54% [51]. These figures were clearly lower for the unfortunate patients exceeding the Milan criteria. The group at Mount Sinai recently published a series of 36 patients undergoing LDLT for HCC, including 21 patients with tumors outside the Milan criteria [52]. Two-year overall survival was 60%. In Japan, a recent multicenter survey including 316 patients undergoing living donor transplant for HCC was reported, with 172 patients beyond the Milan criteria [25]. Median follow-up was short, only 16 months, which results in an underestimation of tumor recurrence. Recurrence was significantly higher (22.2%) in patients with tumors beyond when compared with those within the Milan criteria (1.4%). In addition, 3-year survival was significantly lower for patients outside the Milan criteria when compared with those within the limits (60% versus 79%, respectively). These studies also identify an under/over estimation of the tumor stage prior transplantation ranging between 21% to 63%.

## Summary

Given the current information available, there is no compelling scientific data for expanding the accepted criteria for CLT in HCC. The proposals for expansion are based on explant examination, and up to now, no imaging techniques have been shown to have the same diagnostic accuracy as pathology. If the University from California–San Francisco and Pittsburgh definitions were to be applied to radiologic reports, then we would surely list patients with unidentified more advanced tumor stage in whom understaging would have an impact. These series lack of informative data on dropout rate and intention-to-treat survival and overall survival for the specific group of patients in which the expanded criteria is applied. Only one series of CLT from Mount Sinai reported specific outcomes for patients with expanded criteria (5-year survival: 44%, 5-year intention-to-treat survival: 25%) [43]. As we recently suggested, the proposed expanded tumor stage for LT should perhaps become the criteria for exclusion from the waiting list because of tumor progression [53]. Consequently, making changes to a widely accepted and repeatedly proven criteria, which is the basis of the current organ allocation policy, based on the above data without prospective studies demonstrating good outcomes would be unwise. Results coming from LDLT should be considered aside, and are difficult to extrapolate toward policy decisions for cadaver transplants. A modest expansion of the criteria for LDLT in patients that otherwise will receive locoregional treatments might be considered in the setting of research studies, but not as a consolidated clinical practice.

On the other hand, further refinement of the predictors of recurrence is needed. Vascular invasion, poor differentiation degree, tumor size, and in some studies, bilobar disease, are identified as the major predictors of recurrence. When restricting the selection criteria to patients with early HCC, however, only vascular invasion appears as a predictor of recurrence, if enough number of events in a given series allows this analysis. This marker is associated with some of the recurrences that have occurred in patients with tumors meeting the current Milan criteria (4–17% of the cases). Other factors, such as size or poor tumor differentiation, are indirect surrogates of this predictive marker [54]. Even so, vascular invasion is an imperfect marker of the biologic aggressiveness of HCC. Conversely, some patients with tumors outside of the current limits might not recur, and it seems that there is no "cutoff" below which tumors will not recur, but that rather, there is a continuum along which an increase in the size and number of transplanted tumors will result in a linear increase in the likelihood of recurrence. Ongoing research in the genetic profiling of HCC may provide a more accurate method for stratifying HCC patients according to the risk of recurrent disease [55].

## References

[1] Parkin DM, Bray F, Ferlay J, et al. Estimating the world cancer burden: Globocan 2000. Int J Cancer 2001;94:153–6.

[2] El-Serag HB, Mason AC. Rising incidence of hepatocellular carcinoma in the United States. N Engl J Med 1999;340:745–50.

[3] Sangiovanni A, Del Ninno E, Fasani P, et al. Increased survival of cirrhotic patients with hepatocellular carcinoma detected during surveillance. Gastroenterology 2004;126:1005–14.

[4] Llovet JM, Burroughs A, Bruix J. Hepatocellular carcinoma. Lancet 2003;362:1907–17.

[5] Llovet JM, Bruix J, Gores Gj. Surgical resection versus transplantation for early hepatocellular carcinoma: clues for the best strategy. Hepatology 2000;31:1019–21.

[6] Llovet JM, Fuster J, Bruix J. Intention-to-treat analysis of surgical treatment for early hepatocellular carcinoma: resection versus transplantation. Hepatology 1999;30:1434–40.
[7] Mazzaferro V, Regalia E, Doci R, et al. Liver transplantation for the treatment of small hepatocellular carcinomas in patients with cirrhosis. N Engl J Med 1996;334:693–9.
[8] Arii S, Yamaoka Y, Futagawa S, et al. Results of surgical and nonsurgical treatment for small-sized hepatocellular carcinomas: a retrospective and nationwide survey in Japan. Hepatology 2000;32:1224–9.
[9] Sala M, Llovet JM, Vilana R, et al. Initial response to percutaneous ablation predicts survival in patients with hepatocellular carcinoma. Hepatology 2004;40:1352–60.
[10] Llovet JM, Bruix J. Systematic review of randomized trials for unresectable hepatocellular carcinoma: chemoembolization improves survival. Hepatology 2003;37:429–42.
[11] Llovet JM, Real MI, Montaña X, et al. Arterial embolisation or chemoembolization versus symptomatic treatment in patients with unresectable hepatocellular carcinoma: a randomized controlled trial. Lancet 2002;359:1734–9.
[12] Ringe B, Pichlmayr R, Wittekind C, Tusch G. Surgical treatment of hepatocellular carcinoma: experience with liver resection and transplantation in 198 patients. World J Surg 1991; 15:270–85.
[13] Iwatsuki S, Starzl TE, Sheahan DG, et al. Hepatic resection versus transplantation for hepatocellular carcinoma. Ann Surg 1991;214:221–9.
[14] Bismuth H, Chiche L, Adam R, et al. Liver resection versus transplantation for hepatocellular carcinoma in cirrhotic patients. Ann Surg 1993;218:145–51.
[15] Moreno P, Jaurrieta E, Figueras J, et al. Orthotopic liver transplantation: treatment of choice in cirrhotic patients with hepatocellular carcinoma? Transplant Proc 1995;27:2296–8.
[16] Iwatsuki S, Gordon RD, Shaw BW, Starzl TE. Role of liver transplantation in cancer therapy. Ann Surg 1985;202:401–7.
[17] Llovet JM, Bruix J, Fuster J, et al. Liver transplantation for small hepatocellular carcinoma: the tumor-node-metastasis classification does not have prognostic power. Hepatology 1998;27:1572–7.
[18] Bismuth H, Majno PE, Adam R. Liver transplantation for hepatocellular carcinoma. Semin Liver Dis 1999;19:311–22.
[19] Jonas S, Bechstein WO, Steinmüller T, et al. Vascular invasion and histopathologic grading determine outcome after liver transplantation for hepatocellular carcinoma in cirrhosis. Hepatology 2001;33:1080–6.
[20] Harnois DM, Steers J, Andrews JC, et al. Preoperative hepatic artery chemoembolization followed by orthotopic liver transplantation for hepatocellular carcinoma. Liver Transpl Surg 1999;5:192–9.
[21] Roayaie S, Ben-Haim M, Fishbein TM, et al. Comparison of surgical outcomes for hepatocellular carcinoma in patients with hepatitis B versus hepatitis C: A Western experience. Ann Surg Oncol 2000;7:764–70.
[22] Llovet JM, Sala M, Fuster J, et al. Predictors of drop-out and survival of patients with hepatocellular carcinoma candidates for liver transplantation. Hepatology 2003;38:763A.
[23] Hemming AW, Nelson DR, Reed AI. Liver transplantation for hepatocellular carcinoma. Minerva Chir 2002;57:575–85.
[24] Shetty K, Timmins K, Brensinger C, et al. Liver transplantation for hepatocellular carcinoma validation of present selection criteria in predicting outcome. Liver Transpl 2004;10: 911–8.
[25] Todo S, Furukawa H. Living donor liver transplantation for adult patients with hepatocellular carcinoma: experience in Japan. Ann Surg 2004;240:451–61.
[26] Bruix J, Llovet JM. Prognostic prediction in HCC: did anyone expect it to be easy? Hepatology 2004;39:551–2.
[27] Yao FY, Bass NM, Nikolai B, et al. A follow-up analysis of the pattern and predictors of drop-out from the waiting list for liver transplantation in patients with hepatocellular carcinoma: implications for the current organ allocation policy. Liver Transpl 2003;9:684–92.

[28] Maddala YK, Stadheim L, Andrews JC, et al. Drop-out rates of patients with hepatocellular cancer listed for liver transplantation: outcome with chemoembolization. Liver Transpl 2004;10:449–55.
[29] Herrero JI, Sangro B, Quiroga J, et al. Influence of tumor characteristics on the outcome of liver transplantation among patients with liver cirrhosis and hepatocellular carcinoma. Liver Transpl 2001;7:631–6.
[30] Yao FY, Ferrell L, Bass NM, et al. Liver transplantation for hepatocellular carcinoma: expansion of the tumor size limits does not adversely impact survival. Hepatology 2001;33:1394–403.
[31] Marsh JW, Dvorchik I. Liver organ allocation for hepatocellular carcinoma: are we sure? Liver Transpl 2003;9:693–6.
[32] Cillo U, Vitale A, Bassanello M, et al. Liver transplantation for the treatment of moderately or well-diffrentiated hepatocellular carcinoma. Ann Surg 2004;239:150–9.
[33] Freeman RB, Wiesner RH, Harper A, et al. The new liver allocation system: moving toward evidence-based transplantation policy. Liver Transpl 2002;8:851–8.
[34] Sharma P, Balan V, Hernandez JL, et al. Liver transplantation for hepatocellular carcinoma: the impact of MELD. Liver Transpl 2004;10:36–41.
[35] Majno PE, Adam R, Bismuth H, et al. Influence of preoperative transarterial lipiodol chemoembolization on resection and transplantation for hepatocellular carcinoma in patients with cirrhosis. Ann Surg 1997;226:688–703.
[36] Llovet JM, Mas X, Aponte JJ, et al. Cost effectiveness of adjuvant therapy for hepatocellular carcinoma during the waiting list for liver transplantation. Gut 2002;50:123–8.
[37] Bruix J, Sherman M, Llovet JM, et al. Clinical management of hepatocellular carcinoma. Conclusions of the 2000 EASL conference. J Hepatol 2001;35:421–30.
[38] Murakami T, Mochizuki K, Nakamura H. Imaging evaluation of the cirrhotic liver. Semin Liver Dis 2001;21:213–24.
[39] Rizzi PM, Kane PA, Ryder SD, et al. Accuracy of radiology in detection of hepatocellular carcinoma before liver transplantation. Gastroenterology 1994;107:1425–9.
[40] De Carlis L, Giacomoni A, Pirotta V, et al. Surgical treatment of hepatocellular cancer in the era of hepatic transplantation. J Am Coll Surg 2003;196:887–97.
[41] Burrel M, Llovet JM, Ayuso C, et al. MRI angiography is superior to helical CT for detection of HCC prior to liver transplantation: an explant correlation. Hepatology 2003;38:1034–42.
[42] Teefey SA, Hildebolt CC, Dehdashti F, et al. Detection of primary hepatic malignancy in liver transplant candidates: prospective comparison of CT, MR imaging, US and PET. Radiology 2003;226:533–42.
[43] Roayaie S, Frischer J, Emre SH, et al. Long-term results with multimodal adjuvant therapy and liver transplantation for the treatment of hepatocellular carcinomas larger than 5 cm. Ann Surg 2002;235:533–9.
[44] Steinmüller T, Pascher A, Sauer IM, et al. Living-donation liver transplantation for hepatocellular carcinoma: time to drop the limitations? Transplant Proc 2002;34:2263–4.
[45] Trotter JF, Wachs M, Everson GT, et al. Adult-to-adult transplantation of the right hepatic lobe from a living donor. N Engl J Med 2002;346:1074–82.
[46] Sarasin FP, Majno PE, Llovet JM, et al. Living donor liver transplantation for early hepatocellular carcinoma: a life-expectancy and cost-effectiveness perspective. Hepatology 2001;33:1073–9.
[47] Bozorgzadeh A, Jain A, Ryan C, et al. Impact of hepatitis C viral infection in primary cadaveric liver allograft versus primary living-donor allograft in 100 consecutive liver transplant recipients receiving tacrolimus. Transplantation 2004;77:1066–107.
[48] Garcia-Retortillo M, Forns X, Llovet JM, et al. Hepatitis C recurrence is more severe after living donor transplantation compared to cadaveric liver transplantation. Hepatology 2004; 40:699–707.
[49] Libbrecht L, Bielen D, Verslype C, et al. Focal lesions in cirrhotic explant livers: pathological evaluation and accuracy of pretransplantation imaging examinations. Liver Transpl 2002;8:749–61.

[50] Llovet JM, García-Valdecasas JC, Fuster J, et al. Living donor liver transplantation for hepatocellular carcinoma with explanted criteria: evaluation of applicability in Europe. Liver Transpl 2003;9:C–64 [A].

[51] Kaihara S, Kiuchi T, Ueda M, et al. Living donor liver transplantation for hepatocellular carcinoma. Transplantation 2003;75:S37–40.

[52] Gondolesi G, Roayaie S, Muñoz L, et al. Adult living donor liver transplantation for patients with hepatocellular carcinoma: extending UNOS priority criteria. Ann Surg 2004;239:142–9.

[53] Bruix J, Fuster J, Llovet JM. Liver transplantation for hepatocellular carcinoma: Foucault Pendulum vs evidence-based decision. Liver Transpl 2003;9:700–2.

[54] Schwartz ME. Liver transplantation for hepatocellular carcinoma. Gastroenterology 2004; 127(S1):268–76.

[55] Llovet JM, Wurmbach E. Gene expression profiles in hepatocellular carcinoma: not yet there. J Hepatol 2004;41:336–9.

ELSEVIER
SAUNDERS

Clin Liver Dis 9 (2005) 329–346

CLINICS IN
LIVER DISEASE

# Prevention of Hepatocellular Carcinoma

Antonio Craxì, MD[a,*], Calogero Cammà, MD[a,b]

[a]*Cattedra di Gastroenterologia, University of Palermo, Clinica Medica I, Piazza della Cliniche 2, 90127, Italy*
[b]*IBIM, Consiglio Nazionale delle Ricerche, Palermo, Italy*

Hepatocellular carcinoma (HCC) is a leading cause of morbidity and mortality. Its annual incidence, estimated to be 250,000 to 1,000,000 new cases worldwide, is increasing in industrialized countries, whereas most rates for other cancer are decreasing. Currently, HCC is the fifth most common cancer worldwide and the third most common cause of cancer-related death in males [1]. Estimates on the viral spread time are consistent with epidemiologic observations, and predict that the burden of HCC in hepatitis C virus (HCV) cirrhosis will increase in the next 2 to 3 decades in the United States, possibly to equal that currently experienced in Japan [2].

The extensive application of surveillance programs for early detection of small HCC has increased the number of tumors detected at a subclinical stage, as well as that of lesions potentially responsive to curative treatments [3]. Nonetheless, the 5-year survival rate of patients with small (< 5 cm) HCC undergoing surgical or percutaneous ablation is lower than 50% [4]. This holds true even within intensive screening programs, because of the almost constant presence of underlying cirrhosis and of the high risk of local and distant recurrence, even though treatment had been considered radical. The benefits of orthotopic liver transplantation in patients with small HCC are somewhat limited by the high rate of tumor progression and death due to liver disease while still on the waiting list. This applies even to countries with a high rate of organs available for orthotopic liver transplantation [4].

Although early diagnosis and effective treatments are paramount in controlling the death rate of patients with HCC, the importance of cancer preven-

The full cost of this study was sustained by the institutions for which the authors work.
* Corresponding author.
*E-mail address:* craxanto@unipa.it (A. Craxì).

1089-3261/05/$ – see front matter 
doi:10.1016/j.cld.2004.12.008 **_liver.theclinics.com_**

tion has gradually emerged because advanced (ie, large or locally invasive) HCC is difficult to cure. Because the basic mechanism of all cancer development results from accumulation of epigenetic and genetic alterations in cells, the current concept of multistage carcinogenesis has promoted chemoprevention to the stage of a new medical science [5]. Therefore, HCC (chemo)-prevention remains a major issue in the long-term management of cirrhotic patients, especially where chronic HCV or hepatitis B virus (HBV) infection are the leading cause of chronic liver disease (up to 80% in the Mediterranean area) [6].

Chemoprevention may be defined as the use of natural or synthetic agents to reverse, suppress, or prevent premalignant lesions from progressing to invasive cancer [7]. Chemoprevention of HCC may be classified into three categories: (1) primary, preventing cancer in healthy subjects at high risk for etiologic factors known to cause chronic liver disease; (2) secondary, preventing cancer in those with premalignant conditions, for example, HCC prevention in patients with cirrhosis; (3) tertiary, preventing recurrence in patients cured of an initial cancer.

A prevention program for HCC should fulfill the following prerequisites: (1) identification of the risk factors for HCC; (2) determination of the pathogenetic mechanisms of liver carcinogenesis as well as of the genetic markers that identify the early events in the carcinogenetic process and possibly availability of animal tumor models; and finally, (3) evaluation of the available data from epidemiologic and clinical studies on candidate (chemo) preventive agents.

## High-risk populations

Because treating an entire population with pharmacologic agents to prevent cancer in a few is not the goal of prevention, intensive screening and prevention programs should be confined to patients at high risk of developing HCC. Clinically defined high-risk groups are well known [8]. However, the accuracy and the reliability of recognized clinical, virologic, histologic, and molecular risk factors for neoplastic transformation are still insufficient; thus, accurate risk prediction of developing cancer in individual patients remains an elusive goal. Ideally, information about pathogenetic molecular markers of high HCC risk would be helpful. In these marker-positive individuals, chemoprevention would be cost effective, and might be targeted at the specific locus responsible for the individual's risk.

The geographic distribution of HCC is highly uneven: three geographic areas with different incidence rates (low, intermediate, and high) have been recognized [1,9]. This geographic variability of HCC incidence suggests that one or more risk factors are most prevalent in the areas of higher incidence, but not in areas where the incidence of HCC is less.

HCC development is closely related to chronic inflammation of the liver due to hepatitis viral infections, and most commonly arises in a cirrhotic liver [6]. The annual incidence of HCC reaches approximately 2% to 7% in HBV or HCV cirrhosis [10]. In Europe and the United States, an estimated 20% to 40% of patients with chronic HBV or HCV infection develop cirrhosis within 15 to 30 years, and many of these will develop HCC. Dual HBV and HCV coinfection increases the risk for development of HCC [11]. These projections are important, because approximately 170 million people are infected with HCV and 400 million individuals harboring a chronic HBV infection.

According to a consensus report of the National Institutes of Health, the annual probability of liver cancer among patients with chronic HBV is 0.5%, and that among patients with cirrhosis is 2.4%. Studies on natural history of HBV infection conclusively show that the risk of HCC development increases with age, with the persistence of abnormal aminotransferases and with higher necroinflammation on liver biopsy. Data on the incidence of HCC emerging from longitudinal studies with prolonged follow-up must be considered with caution due to the selection and increased surveillance for cases with more severe disease. There is evidence, from a long-term prospective study by Villa et al [12] in a homogeneous cohort of inactive HBV carriers, that this condition by itself is not associated with a higher risk of HCC in Caucasian subjects. The authors concluded that over a 30-year period, chronic HBV carrier blood donors from Northern Italy did not develop clinically significant liver disease, HCC, or other liver-related morbidity or mortality at a higher rate than uninfected controls. The presence of medical comorbidities, older age at diagnosis, abnormal glutamyltransferase (GGT) levels (surrogate index of alcohol abuse) were independent predictors of death among chronic HBV carriers.

An unknown number of subjects in the general population harbor occult HBV infection, that is, the presence of HBV genomes in the liver in the absence of detectable amounts of hepatitis B surface antigen (HBsAg) and even of any other marker of HBV infection in the blood [13]. This condition is found in more than 50% of subjects with chronic HCV infection in highly endemic areas, possibly due to the common pathways of spread of HBV and HCV. In this context, occult HBV infection may be related to a high risk of carcinogenesis in HCV cirrhosis [14].

Actually, in a recent study [15] investigating the prevalence and molecular status of occult HBV in 107 patients with HCC and 192 patients with chronic hepatitis, all HCV-RNA positive and HBsAg negative in serum, occult HBV-DNA was detected in the liver of 68 cases of HCC (63.5%) and in 63 of chronic hepatitis (32.8%) ($P < 0.0001$; odds ratio [OR], 3.6; 95% confidence interval [CI], 2.2–5.9). The significant association of occult HBV with HCC was irrespective of age and sex. However, further prospective studies may prove useful to substantiate this association.

Cirrhosis per se is a precancerous condition, but the magnitude of the oncogenic risk varies widely with etiology, that is, high with HBV and HCV and low with alcohol [16]. Large and small cell dysplasia have been held to be associated with an increased risk of malignant change for many years, especially in studies from Africa, Italy, and France, and macroregenerative nodules, adenomatous hyperplasia, dysplastic nodules (synonyms denoting large cirrhotic nodules with cytologic and architectural abnormalities) in Japan and the United States. Both suggestions have generated debate, and neither can be regarded as obligatory steps in carcinogenesis because they are not seen in noncirrhotic livers with HCC.

## Putative understanding of molecular mechanisms of liver carcinogenesis

Hepatic carcinogenesis has been extensively investigated in experimental animals, mainly by the use of chemicals. These studies established the multistep nature of malignant transformation through initiation, promotion, and progression. The findings are now increasingly applied to humans. However, only fragmentary and incomplete data are available, and the pathogenesis of HCC remains poorly defined [17].

The development of molecular genetic and cytogenetic approaches has given rise to information on the overall pattern of chromosomal aberrations in HCC, showing both common features with other neoplasms and specific traits. Although some common genetic abnormalities, such as loss of tumor suppressors p53 and p16, have been reported, the absence of an obviously inherited predisposition to liver cancer has hampered the identification of critical genes located in many candidate chromosomal regions, precluding an orderly overview of the rate-limiting steps involved in multistage hepatocarcinogenesis.

Furthermore, current knowledge about molecular pathogenesis of HCC is a result of investigations of fully developed HCC, and much less is known about the genetic basis of preneoplastic lesions or predisposing conditions (ie, chronic hepatitis, cirrhosis macroregenerative nodules, dysplastic nodules). This, in fact, is the most critical issue to be addressed to get a clear picture of progression of HCC from its precursors and to identify gene markers for delimiting cancers from noncancerous lesions. Additional effort needs to be focused on identification of molecular changes during the evolution of HCC. There are only a few correlations between genetic alterations and clinicopathologic parameters, including molecular basis of metastatic potentials, recurrence, and responsiveness to therapy. Continuing studies of the relationship between genetic alterations and hepatocarcinogenesis are needed to identify critical regulatory pathways involved in molecular pathogenesis of HCC.

## Primary prevention

In the setting of primary prevention the epidemiologic data available point to vaccination against HBV as the most efficient primary prevention measure currently available to reduce the HCC incidence and mortality in high-incidence areas. Eradication of HBV by vaccination has reduced the incidence of HCC in children in Taiwan [18], becoming the most radical way to prevent HCC associated with chronic HBV.

Because vaccination against HCV is yet unavailable and there is only a low probability of a vaccine against HCV being developed in the near future, other preventive methods are required to reduce the burden of HCV-related liver disease (Fig. 1). Primary prevention of new infection by rigorous implementation of infection control practice to prevent nosocomial and iatrogenic HCV transmission and secondary prevention of HCV transmission from infected persons to other persons through counselling are needed [19]. However, the impact of any prevention program on HCV spread is relatively low because the majority of the infected patients are not under medical care. Although screening of the whole population is not recommended, it is important to test for HCV all persons with risk factors for HCV infection.

A strategy aiming at preventing chronic liver disease of any etiology (alcohol, obesity, others) may be required to prevent HCC in low- and intermediate-incidence areas, and hence, worldwide. The incidence of HCC might be further reduced by eliminating aflatoxin from the food supply in areas of the world where agricultural products are stored under conditions that favor the growth of *Aspergillus flavus* and *Aspergillus parasiticus*. A recent case–control study conducted in Sudan clearly demonstrated that reduction of aflatoxin contamination of foods may be useful public health strategy in HCC prevention [20].

Only well-recognized risk factors for HCC were dealt with in this paragraph. Others risk factors, like anabolic or sex steroids, smoking habits, and perhaps plant-derived or chemical agents have not been considered, because their impact on HCC epidemiology is doubtful or very small, and available data are sparse and somewhat conflicting.

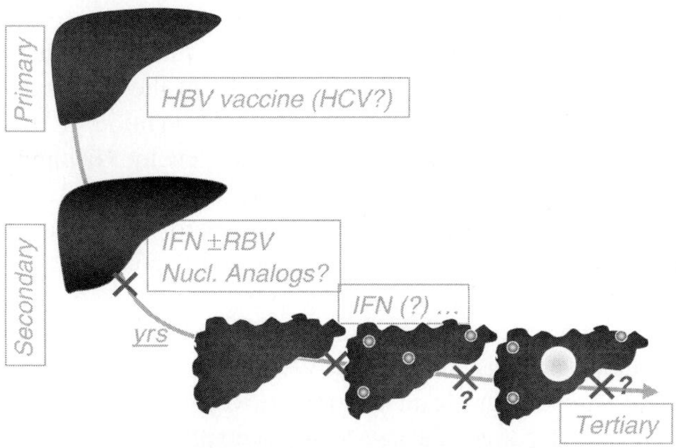


Fig. 1. Prevention programs for HCC from viral etiology.

## Secondary prevention

### *Interferon for hepatitis C virus cirrhosis*

It has been argued that long-term suppression of viral replication could reduce hepatocyte turnover and lessen the risk of dysplasia and cancer. In 1995, a small randomized controlled trial (RCT) showed a decrease in the incidence of HCC in patients with HCV cirrhosis compared with untreated controls [21]. On the wake of this study, several controlled trials [22–41] were performed, mostly in patients with HCV infection. These studies, often assessing retrospectively collected cohorts of a relatively small size and showed a marked degree of heterogeneity, making it difficult to assess the actual level of benefit obtained by interferon (IFN) treatment.

Hitherto, a number of important questions still remain unsolved by the available studies: Is the risk of HCC in viral cirrhosis reduced by IFN therapy? If a risk reduction truly exists, does the benefit apply to all patients with HCV or HBV cirrhosis? Is a sustained response to IFN required to reduce the HCC incidence? Does the preventive effect of IFN on HCC development starts before the onset of severe fibrosis or cirrhosis?

We have updated to the current date a previous systematic overview of the available literature [42] to evaluate whether IFN reduces the incidence of HCC in patients with viral cirrhosis. The effect of IFN on cancer incidence (three RCTs and 17 NRCTs: 4659 patients) is shown in Fig. 2. IFN seemingly decreased HCC rate in all but one of 20 evaluable studies, a significant difference being observed in 13. The pooled estimate of the treatment effect was significantly in favor of a preventive effectiveness of IFN (risk difference [RD], −12.2; CI, −8.4 to −16.1, $P<0.00001$).

We found a remarkable heterogeneity among the studies ($\chi^2$ for heterogeneity 69.1 with 19 *df*; $P<0.0001$). The most prominent heterogeneity was in the difference of magnitude of the treatment effect on the risk of cancer ("quantitative heterogeneity"). Large differences were observed in the baseline risk of HCC among the different trials: the HCC rate in the untreated group ranged from 6.8% to 73%. These two trials represent the extremes of the range of effectiveness: Sofia found no effect of IFN on prevention of HCC, while the highest preventive benefit of treatment was observed by Nishiguchi [21]. The small sample size of the latter study could be the result of unbalanced randomization. This is suggested by the low cancer rate in the treated group (26% %) and by the extremely high cancer rate in the control group (73%). RD of each trial ranged from −33.3% [41] to +3.9% [43]. A pooled analysis excluding both outliers reporting the highest [21] and lowest [29] benefit of IFN yelded once more inconsistent results. We searched for the sources of this variability and found a significant relation between the IFN benefit and HCC rate among untreated patients using both parametric and nonparametric tests (Pearson coefficient, r = −0.77, $P$ = 0.0001; Spearman rank correlation coefficient, r = −0.74, $P$ = 0.0001).

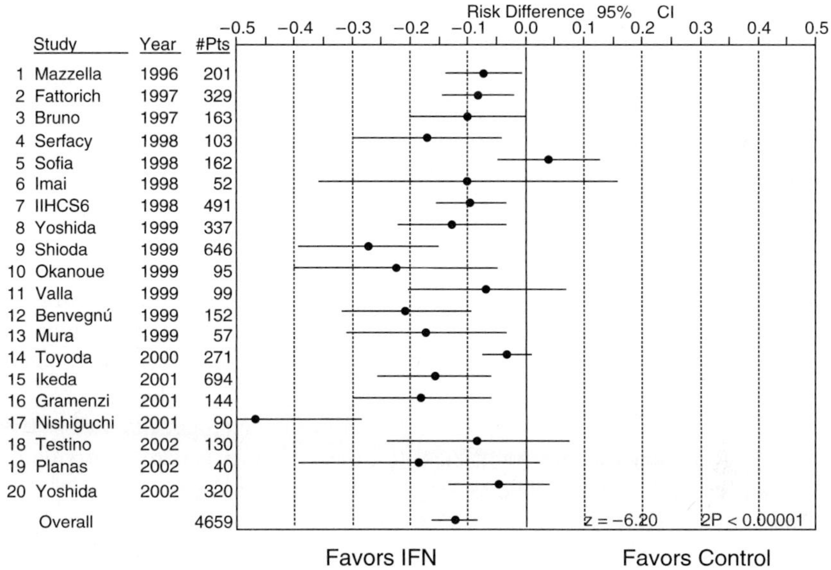


Fig. 2. Meta-analysis of the 20 controlled trials of IFN for prevention of HCC in patients with HCV-related cirrhosis. RD and 95% CI for each study and the pooled estimate of the treatment effect with its CI are plotted on the graph. Studies are arranged by publication year.

Because the 20 studies show a marked heterogeneity, subgroup analyses were performed in relation to the different design (RCTs versus NRCTs), ethnic origin of patients (European versus Oriental studies), HCC incidence in the untreated group (rate in controls $\geq 20\%$ versus $< 20\%$) and type of publication (full papers versus abstracts). Consistent results were only observed when assessing data pooled from RCTs, European reports, studies published as full papers, and from trials where HCC frequency among untreated patients was lower than 20% during the follow-up period, ranging between 32 and 76 months.

To test whether the difference in HCC incidence between treated and untreated groups persisted after adjustment for potentially relevant confounding factors, we performed a logistic regression model including IFN treatment, length of follow-up, cancer rate among untreated patients, design of study (RCTs versus NRCTs), type of publication, and ethnic origin of patients. The final model shows cirrhotic patients treated with IFN have a lower likelihood of developing HCC (OR, 0.28), after adjusting for covariates. Separate subanalyses were performed to evaluate any possible evidence of differential benefit on HCC prevention according to biochemical response to IFN. Analysis by response to treatment showed the pooled RD was −19.1% (CI, −13.1 to −25.2, $P < 0.00001$) among sustained biochemical responders, without a significant heterogeneity ($\chi^2$ for heterogeneity 15.35, $P = 0.053$). The number needed to treat (NNT), evaluated studies including those with consistent results only, is 10.

When only patients from these studies who had a sustained response were evaluated, the NNT dropped to 5.2.

To assess whether the preventive effect of IFN on HCC development is independent from the presence of cirrhosis, we analyzed the results of four other studies [32,39–41], which assess cohorts of subjects with noncirrhotic chronic hepatitis. They included a total of 4011 patients with biopsy-proven chronic hepatitis without cirrhosis at the time of IFN therapy start or during follow-up. One hundred forty-one patients developed HCC over a mean follow-up ranging between 52 and 62 months. We assessed the difference in the rate of HCC between sustained responders and nonsustained responders. IFN significantly decreased the rate of HCC in all studies, independently fron the presence of cirrhosis but proportionally to the degree of fibrosis before tretment. The pooled estimate of the preventive effect of IFN was significant (RD, −4.1%, 95% CI, −2.5 to −5.5, $P < 0.00001$), without significant heterogeneity ($\chi^2 = 0.89$, $P = 0.83$). Reported data are insufficient to assess whether patients evolving into HCC had also developed cirrhosis after the pretreatment assessment.

The results of this meta-analysis demonstrate that the heterogeneity in the magnitude of the preventive effect of IFN on the risk of cancer is the most impressive feature of these studies. This inconsistency among trials is not surprising, because of potential biases in patients selection and in their allocation to treatment groups. It is also evident that studies with high HCC rates among controls are more likely to demonstrate a higher estimate of treatment efficacy, whereas those with low rates are more likely to show no benefit.

Regarding HCV cirrhosis, the pooled data suggested a slight preventive effect of IFN on HCC development in patients with HCV cirrhosis. The magnitude of this effect was low, and the observed benefit might be due to spurious associations. The preventive effect was more evident among sustained biochemical responders to IFN, which intrinsically represent a small proportion of all cirrhotic patients.

### *Interferon for hepatitis B virus cirrhosis*

IFN has been the mainstay of therapy for chronic HBV since the early 1980s. Since then, several RCTs and cohort studies have been published. The results of these trials remain inconsistent about the natural history of HBV disease, because the overall assessment of treatment effect on true disease end points (ie, progression to cirrhosis, to HCC, and death) cannot usually be assessed in short-term trials [44]. A major issue of concern is the fact that RCTs of IFN for chronic HBV have been mostly performed in patients without advanced fibrosis or cirrhosis. The transferability of results to the whole spectrum of subjects with chronic liver disease due to HBV is, hence, questionable.

Long-term retrospective or prospective studies to evaluate the benefits of IFN therapy on HCC chemoprevention will also be difficult to perform due to the prolonged and slow course of the disease. Moreover, no further prospective cohort studies on the course of untreated disease will be feasible because IFN is widely used for the treatment of chronic HBV.

We reviewed and update here our previous meta-analyses [45] of the available literature, to estimate wether IFN reduces the incidence of HCC in HBV cirrhosis. Potentially relevant papers were initially classified into two subsets (1: controlled trials; 2: cohort studies).

*Subset 1 (controlled trials)*

The rate of HCC in treated and untreated patients with HBV cirrhosis was reported in 11 studies [22,25,30,35–38,46–48], including 2560 patients. The benefit of IFN on cancer development is shown in Fig. 3. IFN seemingly decreased the rate of HCC in all but one trial, while a significant difference was observed in three studies. The pooled estimate of the preventive effect of treatment was significantly in favor of IFN (RD, −4.1; 95% CI, −0.8 to −7, $P<0.013$). A remarkable heterogeneity was detected among studies ($\chi^2$ for heterogeneity: 39.12 with 10 *df*; $P = 0.0001$).

Because the 11 trials showed significant inconsistency, subgroup analyses were performed in relation to the ethnic origin of patients (European versus Oriental studies). Consistent results were only observed when assessing data pooled from European reports: in this subgroup, no preventive effect of HCC was shown.

*Subset 2 (cohort studies)*

It has been suggested from long-term cohort studies that IFN treatment may have a protective effect against HCC development in patients with chronic HBV infection. We reviewed the clinical course and outcome of patients enrolled in

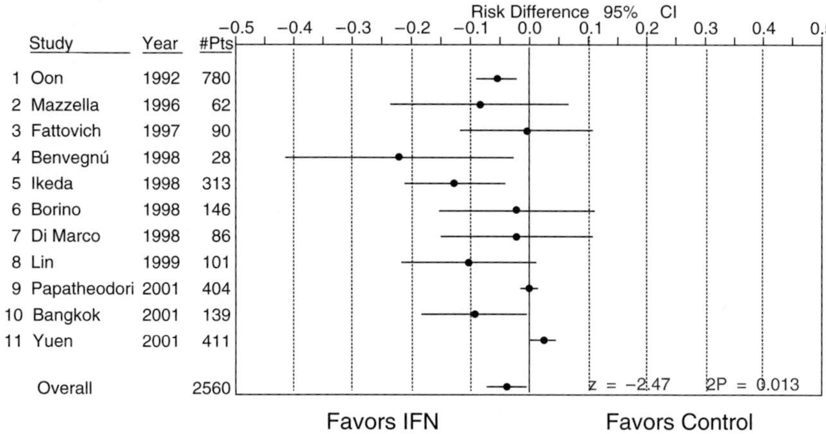


Fig. 3. Meta-analysis of the 11 controlled trials of IFN for prevention of HCC in patients with HBV-related cirrhosis. RD and 95% CI for each study and the pooled estimate of the treatment effect with its CI are plotted on the graph. Studies are arranged by publication year.

long term follow-up studies [47–57]. The 12 studies (11 prospective and one retrospective) included a total of 1952 patients, 1187 not receiving active treatment. Length of follow-up ranged from 2.1 to 8.9 years (mean 6.1). Meta-analysis of longitudinal studies with prolonged follow-up (Fig. 4) showed no significat differences in the rate of HCC between treated patients (1.9%; 95% CI, 0.8–3.0%) and controls (3.16%; 95% CI, 1.8–4.5%).

All the data on HCC development and on liver-related mortality coming from studies with prolonged follow-up must be interpreted with caution, because possible biases can lead to erroneous estimates: (1) data collected from both prospective and retrospective studies conducted in tertiary care centers with limited generalizability; (2) lack of randomization reducing the internal and the external validity of the studies; (3) heterogeneity of patients enrolled, both in respect of clinical and demographic features and of possible cofactors; (4) slow and prolonged course of the disease not allowing an inception cohort; (5) few clinically relevant events, relatively small sample size, and duration of follow-up less than 8 to 10 years; (6) high mortality from nonhepatic causes; (7) selection and increased surveillance for cases with more severe disease and unfavorable course; (8) progressive shift over the years of the global spectrum of the disease due to intervening factors (eg, new diagnostic tests and screening programs; new treatments).

The available evidence of the studies in HBV cirrhosis is less encouraging compared with data obtained in HCV cirrhosis. Studies show a strong heterogeneity, which makes the reliability of conclusions of individual trials questionable. This inconsistency disappeared when the Asian studies were excluded from the analysis, making the overall preventive effect of IFN not significant. On this basis, there is not firm ground to recommend IFN to prevent HCC in

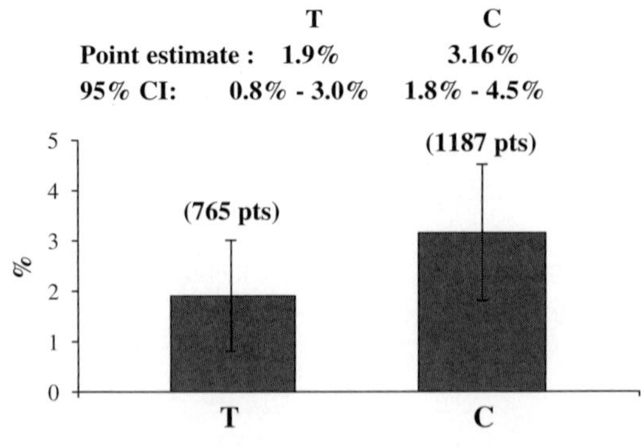


Fig. 4. Probability distribution of development of HCC rate in HBeAg-positive chronic HBV from IFN treated (T) and controls (C). Data from cohort studies. (Reproduced with permission from Craxì A, Di Bona D, Cammà C. Interferon-α for HBeAg positive chronic hepatitis B. J Hepatol 2003;39:S99–105).

HBV cirrhosis. Obviously, IFN-induced viral clearance remains a major outcome for patients with HBV chronic liver disease and indirectly reduces the risk of cancer. Some cases of HBV-associated HCC are observed in the absence of cirrhosis (mostly young males with perinatal infection), and have a very aggressive clinical course. No information on the effectiveness of IFN in preventing this subtype of HCC can be gathered from the available studies.

Even though no serologic evidence of HBV infection is present, occult HBV genomes can be found in the liver of subjects with chronic HCV [30], and could favor neoplastic transformation. Data from one of the studies in our meta-analysis [25] highlight serology of HBV infection (anti-HBc positivity) as an additional risk factor for cancer development in HCV cirrhosis. In this report, the protective effect of IFN was much stronger in anti-HCV–positive patients who did not have a (supposed) occult HBV infection. Although interesting and biologically sound, this approach requires further confirmation through biomolecular techniques able to identify the actual presence of HBV genomes in these patients before translating into practice any recommendation about the preventive use of IFN.

In conclusion, regarding HBV cirrhosis, there is no sound evidence from trials and prospective cohort studies to support a recommendation for widespread use of IFN to prevent HCC in these patients. IFN treatment could help to delay or prevent disease decompensation and liver-related deaths, but further large-scale, multicenter longitudinal studies are needed to prove this point.

### *Lamivudine for HBV cirrhosis*

Lamivudine has a strong and long-lasting inhibitory effect on HBV replication, limited only by the occurrence of drug-resistent mutants [58]. Its effects have mostly been evaluated on surrogate end points such as viral replicative markers and biochemical and histologic indexes of necroinflammation. In this context, lamivudine is highly effective in reducing HBV replication and the short-term progression of liver disease. It is still unclear whether its continuous use in cirrhotic patients might in the long term lessen the rate of occurrence of HCC. Two studies of long-term follow-up are available.

The first [59] compared 436 lamivudine-treated Asian patients (median therapy 32 months, range 0–42) with 215 untreated cases. HBeAg was present at randomization in 58% of these patients. All had an Ishak fibrosis score $\geq 4$. Hepatocellular carcinoma occurred in 17 treated (3.9%) and 16 untreated patients (7.4%) (hazard ratio, 0.49 [0.25–0.99], $P = 0.047$). On average, after 36 months 10% of untreated patients and 5% of those on lamivudine had developed HCC. Among patients on lamivudine, the rate of occurrence of HCC was similar regardless of the occurrence of YMDD drug-resistent mutants (3.6% weight, 4.2% mutant).

The second study [60] has been performed as a retrospective assessment of a cohort of 656 anti-HBe–positive, HBV-DNA–positive Italian patients on long-term lamivudine, 54% with chronic epatitis, and 46% with cirrhosis. On therapy (median 22 months, range 1–66) HBV-DNA suppression was obtained in 616 patients (93.9%). The rate of sustained virological suppression was 39% after 4 years. Thirty-one patients (4.7%) developed HCC during follow-up. Four of them had chronic hepatitis and 27 had cirrhosis before starting lamivudine. The overall incidence of HCC among cirrhotic patients was 4.6%, 8.7%, 19.8%, and 22.1% at 1, 2, 3, and 4 years of therapy. The likelihood of developing HCC was significantly less for cirrhotic patients with sustained virologic suppression ($P < 0.001$), but related to manteinance of the virologic effect of lamivudine. Cox regression analysis indicated that patients with virologic breakthrough had a relative risk of about 3 for HCC development compared with patients with sustained virologic suppression.

Thus, the available experience with lamivudine, the only analog that has been on the market long enough to allow an assessment of long-term efficacy, indicate that a chemopreventive effect on HCC can be reached by its long-term use. There is still no consensus, however, on the need for a protracted virologic response to the drug. Further experience with newer nucleoside/nucleotide analogs such as adefovir is still lacking.

## Tertiary prevention

The 3-year survival rate of patients with liver cancer undergoing percutaneous or surgical treatment remains low, because of the high risk of recurrence even though treatment has been considered curative. A plateau in the effectiveness of ablative treatment (surgical or percutaneous) may well have been reached, and further improvement in survival from a single-modality approach seems unlikely.

Cammà et al [61] followed a large cohort (more then 200) of patients with small ($\leq 5$ cm) HCC in compensated cirrhosis treated by radiofrequency thermal ablation, reported that the 3-year occurrence rate of new lesions was 34%, quite similar to that of a previous study on percutaneous ethanol injection (PEI) (41%) of the same group [62], as well as similat to that found in the study by Lencioni [63], in which the 2-year recurrence rate of patients treated by radiofrequency thermal ablation was 36%. Therefore, all these data underscores, from a practical point of view, the need for adjuvant therapy in the effort to prolong survival and reduce recurrence rates.

The anticancer drugs currently administered for the treatment of unresectable HCC are poorly tolerated in most cases [64], and the fact that the majority of patients will not benefit from therapy highlights the urgent and ongoing need for more effective and safe adjuvant agents. Recently, new agents have been evaluated for adjuvant therapy (tertiary prevention) of HCC recurrence, including retinoids [65], intraarterial I131 [66], adoptive immunotherapy [67], and IFN [68].

*Interferon*

The potential activity of IFN in the setting of secondary chemoprevention has led to the treatment of patients with IFN in the adjuvant setting. Since the first RCT of IFN adjuvant therapy appeared in 2000 [68], four other RCTs have been published [69–72]. Studies have indicated that IFN decreases the rate of cancer recurrence, and the results of our meta-analysis, totaling 196 patients, consistently show a statistically significant benefit on HCC recurrence. The effect of adjuvant IFN treatment on recurrence of HCC is show in Fig. 5. IFN was superior to no treatment in all trials, reaching statistical significance in all but one study. The pooled estimate of the treatment effect was significantly in favor of a beneficial effect of IFN on HCC recurrence (RD, −43%; 95% CI, −65% to −20%, $P<0.0001$). No significant heterogeneity was found among the five trials. The NNT, the number of patients with HCC receving potentially curative treatments needed to treat with IFN to prevent one cancer recurrence is 2.3. However, the key clinical question is whether all patients with HCC receving potentially curative treatments should treat with IFN or whether adjuvant treatment should be administered only to a selected group of patients who clearly stand to benefit. Unfortunately, there is no reliable predoctive model able to identify patient with HCC receving potentially curative treatments and high risk of developing HCC recurrence. Finally, the results of published RCTs remain inconsistent for survival. Further large-scale multicenter RCTs may prove useful to evaluate the benefit on overall survival.

*Acyclic retinoids*

Retinoids, acting on nuclear receptors, retinoic acid receptor (RAR) and retinoid X receptor (RXR) have potential for cancer chemoprevention through their action as regulators of cell growth and differentiation [73].

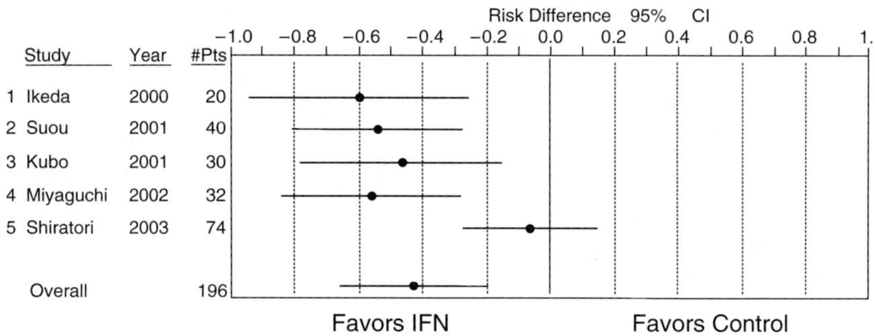


Fig. 5. Meta-analysis of the five controlled trials of IFN for prevention of HCC recurrence in patients with viral cirrhosis and HCC treated with surgical resection or percutaneous ablation. RD and 95% CIs for each study and the pooled estimate of the treatment effect with its CI are plotted on the graph. Studies are arranged by publication year.

Retinoids may inhibit or reverse the carcinogenic process in various types of neoplasms, including the liver, in experimental models of oncogenesis. A preventive approach to HCC by a synthetic retinoid analog, acyclic retinoid, has theoretical interest, because posttranslational modification of RXR by phosphorylation impairs its function, leading to uncontrolled hepatocyte growth. In vitro acyclic retinoid suppress the phosphorylation of RXR α, restores its function in the presence of its endogenous ligand, 9-cis RAR, and thereby induces apoptosis of the cancer cells. HCC in cirrhotic patients contains lower levels of endogenous retinoids, and may be insensitive to retinoic acid because of a malfunction of nuclear retinoid X receptor α (RXRα) [73]. In HCC tissues, there is an accumulation of phospho-inactivated RXRα, which functions as a dominant negative receptor and interferes with transactivation by remaining normal RXRα. Acyclic retinoid prevents phosphorylation of RXRα and restores its function and enhances the sensitivity of HCC cells to IFNs-α and -β, thereby promoting apoptosis induced by these interferons. This could lead to eradication of (pre)malignant clones ("clonal deletion") from the cirrhotic liver.

Clinical use of polyprenoic acid, an orally absorbable acyclic retinoid, has been exploited in the context of tertiary prevention of HCC recurrence after surgical or PEI tumor ablation in 89 cirrhotics [74] . Treatment with polyprenoic acid significantly reduced the incidence of recurrent or new hepatomas. After a median follow-up of 38 months, 12 patients in the polyprenoic acid group (27%) had recurrent or new hepatomas compared with 22 patients in the placebo group (49%, $P = 0.04$). These promising results still await confirmation by other controlled studies.

## Summary

The accuracy and the reliability of well-recognized clinical, virologic, histologic, and molecular risk factors for HCC are still insufficient; thus, accurate risk prediction of developing cancer in individual patients remains an elusive goal.

Future directions in chemprevention of HCC will be on the development of molecular risk models and of new chemopreventive agents. The design of targeted molecular therapies may need to be tailored to the specific molecular phenotype of a specific HCC. Studies examining multiple genes and proteins (genomics and proteomics) in the same HCCs will be required to evaluate this possibility thoroughly.

In the setting of primary prevention, the epidemiologic data available point to vaccination against HBV as the most efficient primary prevention measure currently available to reduce the HCC incidence and mortality in high-incidence areas. A strategy aiming at preventing chronic liver disease of any etiology (HCV infection, alcohol, obesity, others) may be required to prevent HCC in low- and intermediate-incidence areas, and hence, worldwide.

In the setting of secondary chemoprevention, literature data pooling suggest a slight preventive effect of IFN on HCC development in patients with HCV-related cirrhosis. The magnitude of this effect is low, and the observed benefit might be due to spurious associations. The preventive effect is more evident among sustained responders to IFN. There is no sound evidence to support a recommendation for widespread use of IFN to prevent HCC in HBV-related cirrhosis.

In the setting of tertiary chemoprevention, the risk of recurrence of HCC is reduced by IFN treatment in selected patients populations. Further large-scale multicenter RCTs may prove useful to evaluate the benefit on overall survival.

## Acknowledgments

We are indebted to Professor Erica Villa, MD, and Filippo Schepis, MD, for helpful discussion and insight.

## References

[1] Parkin DM, Bray F, Ferlay J, et al. Estimating the world cancer burden: GLOBOCAN 2000. Int J Cancer 2001;94:153–6.
[2] Tanaka Y, Hanada K, Mizokami M, et al. Inaugural Article: a comparison of the molecular clock of hepatitis C virus in the United States and Japan predicts that hepatocellular carcinoma incidence in the United States will increase over the next two decades. Proc Natl Acad Sci USA 2002;99:15584–9.
[3] Yuen MF, Cheng CC, Lauder IJ, et al. Early detection of hepatocellular carcinoma increases the chance of treatment: Hong Kong experience. Hepatology 2000;31:330–5.
[4] Llovet JM, Burroughs A, Bruix J. Hepatocellular carcinoma. Lancet 2003;362:1907–17.
[5] Lippman SM, Hong WK. Cancer prevention by delay. Commentary re: J.A. O'Shaughnessy et al. Treatment and prevention of intraepithelial neoplasia: an important target for accelerated new agent development. Clin Cancer Res 2002;8:305–13.
[6] Stroffolini T, Sagnelli E, Almasio P, et al. Italian Hospitals Collaborating Groups. Characteristics of liver cirrhosis in Italy: results from a multicenter national study. Dig Liver Dis 2004;36:56–60.
[7] Sporn MB, Dunlop NM, Newton DL, et al. Prevention of chemical carcinogenesis by vitamin A and its synthetic analogs (retinoids). Fed Proc 1976;35:1332–8 [review].
[8] Tsukuma H, Hiyama T, Tanaka S, et al. Risk factors for hepatocellular carcinoma among patients with chronic liver disease. N Engl J Med 1993;24(328):1797–801.
[9] Simonetti RG, Camma C, Fiorello F, et al. Hepatocellular carcinoma. A worldwide problem and the major risk factors. Dig Dis Sci 1991;36:962–72 [review].
[10] El-Serang HB, Mason AC. Rising incidence of hepatocellular carcinoma in the United States. N Engl J Med 1999;340:745–50.
[11] Donato F, Boffetta P, Puoti M. A meta-analysis of epidemiological studies on the combined effect of hepatitis B and C virus infections in causing hepatocellular carcinoma. Int J Cancer 1998;75(3):347–54.
[12] Manno M, Cammà C, Schepis F, et al. Natural history of chronic HBV carriers in Northern Italy: morbidity and mortality after 30 years. Gastroenterology 2004;127:756–63.
[13] Torbenson M, Thomas DL. Occult hepatitis B. Lancet Infect Dis 2002;2:479–86.

[14] Cacciola I, Pollicino T, Squadrito G, et al. Occult hepatitis B virus infection in patients with chronic hepatitis C liver disease. N Engl J Med 1999;341:22–6.
[15] Pollicino T, Squadrito G, Cerenzia G, et al. Hepatitis B virus maintains its pro-oncogenic properties in the case of occult HBV infection. Gastroenterology 2004;126:102–10.
[16] Simonetti RG, Camma C, Fiorello F, et al. Hepatitis C virus infection as a risk factor for hepatocellular carcinoma in patients with cirrhosis. A case-control study. Ann Intern Med 1992;116:97–102.
[17] Grisham JW. Molecular genetic alterations in primary hepatocellular neoplasms: hepatocellular adenoma, hepatocellular carcinoma, and hepatoblastoma. In: Coleman WB, Tsongalis GJ, editors. The molecular basis of human cancer. Totowa (NJ): Humana Press; 2001. p. 269–346.
[18] Kao JH, Chen DS. Global control of hepatitis B virus infection. Lancet Infect Dis 2002;2: 395–403.
[19] Kew M, Francois G, Lavanchy D, et al, Viral Hepatitis Prevention Board. Prevention of hepatitis C virus infection. J Viral Hepat 2004;11:198–205 [review].
[20] Omer RE, Kuijsten A, Kadaru AM, et al. Population-attributable risk of dietary aflatoxins and hepatitis B virus infection with respect to hepatocellular carcinoma. Nutr Cancer 2004;48: 15–21.
[21] Nishiguchi S, Kuroki T, Nakatani S, et al. Randomised trial of effects of interferon-α on incidence of hepatocellular carcinoma in chronic active hepatitis C with cirrhosis. Lancet 1995;346:1051–5.
[22] Mazzella G, Accogli E, Sottili S, et al. Alpha-interferon treatment may prevent hepatocellular carcinoma in HCV-related liver cirrhosis. J Hepatol 1996;24:141–7.
[23] Bruno S, Silini E, Crosignani A, et al. Hepatitis C virus genotypes and risk of hepatocellular carcinoma in cirrhosis: a prospective study. Hepatology 1997;25:754–8.
[24] Fattovich G, Giustina G, Degos F, et al. Morbidity and mortality in compensated cirrhosis type C: a retrospective follow-up study of 384 patients. Gastroenterology 1997;112:463–72.
[25] International Interferon-alpha Hepatocellular Carcinoma Study Group. Effect of interferon-alpha on progression of cirrhosis to hepatocellular carcinoma: a retrospective cohort study. Lancet 1998;351:1535–9.
[26] Imai Y, Kawata S, Tamura S, et al, for the Osaka Hepatocellular Carcinoma Prevention Study Group. Relation of interferon therapy and hepatocellular carcinoma in patients with chronic hepatitis C. Ann Intern Med 1998;129:94–9.
[27] Gramenzi A, Andreone P, Fiorino S, et al. Impact of interferon therapy on the natural history of HCV-related cirrhosis. Gut 2001;48:843–8.
[28] Serfaty L, Aumaître H, Cazouillères O, et al. Determinants of outcome of compensated hepatitis C virus-related cirrhosis. Hepatology 1998;27:1435–40.
[29] Sofia S, Casali A, Buscarini E, et al. Effect of lymphoblastoid IFN in the treatment of liver cirrhosis and prevention of HCC. Ital J Gastroenterol Hepatol 1998;30:A31.
[30] Benvegnù L, Chemello L, Noventa F, et al. Retrospective analysis of the effect of interferon therapy on the clinical outcome of patients with viral cirrhosis. Cancer 1998;83:901–9.
[31] Shioda A, Moriyama M, Kaneko M, et al. Long-term prognosis of hepatocellular carcinoma developing after treatment of interferon in patients with chronic hepatitis C and liver cirrhosis. Hepatology 1999;30:268A.
[32] Yoshida H, Shiratori Y, Moriyama M, et al, for the IHIT Study Group. Interferon therapy reduces the risk for hepatocellular carcinoma: national surveillance program of cirrhotic and noncirrhotic patients with chornic hepatitis C in Japan. Ann Intern Med 1999;131:174–81.
[33] Mura D, Deliperi R, Fastame L, et al. Five year follow-up after Interferon therapy in HCV-positive compensated cirrhosis. Ital J Gastroenterol Hepatol 1998;30:A114.
[34] Valla D-C, Chevallier M, Marcellin P, et al. Treatment of hepatitis C virus-related cirrhosis: a randomized controlled trial of interferon alfa 2b versus no treatment. Hepatology 1999; 29:1870–5.
[35] Oon CJ. Long-term survival following treatment of hepatocellular carcinoma in Singapore. Cancer Chemother Pharmacol 1992;31(Suppl):S137–42.

[36] Fattovich G, Giustina G, Realdi G, et al, and the European Concerted Action on Viral Hepatitis (EUROHEP). Long-term outcome of hepatitis B e antigen-positive patients with compensated cirrhosis treated with interferon alfa. Hepatology 1997;26:1338–42.
[37] Di Marco V, Lo Iacono O, Cammà C, et al. The long term course of chronic hepatitis B. Hepatology 1999;30:257–64.
[38] Ikeda K, Saitoh S, Suzuki Y, et al. Interferon decreases hepatocellular carcinogenesis in patients with cirrhosis caused by the hepatitis B virus. Cancer 1998;82:827–35.
[39] Kasahara A, Hayashi N, Mochizuki K, et al. Risk factors for hepatocellular carcinoma and its incidence after interferon treatment in patients with chronic hepatitis C. Hepatology 1998; 27:1394–402.
[40] Cammà C, Di Marco V, Lo Iacono O, et al. Long-term course of interferon-treated chornic hepatitis C. J Hepatol 1998;28:531–7.
[41] Miyajima I, Sata M, Kumashiro R, et al. The incidence of hepatocellular carcinoma in patients with chronic hepatitis C after interferon treatment. Oncol Rep 1998;5:201–4.
[42] Cammà C, Giunta M, Andreone P, et al. Interferon and prevention of hepatocellular carcinoma in viral cirrhosis: an evidence-based approach. J Hepatol 2001;34:593–602.
[43] Fattovich G, Giustina G, Realdi G, et al. Long-term outcome of hepatitis B e antigen-positive patients with compensated cirrhosis treated with interferon alfa. European Concerted Action on Viral Hepatitis (EUROHEP). Hepatology 1997;26:1338–42.
[44] Almasio P, Cammà C, Giunta M, et al. Treatment of chronic hepatitis B: an evidence-based review. In: McDonald JWD, Burroughs A, Feagan BG, editors. Evidence-based gastroenterology and hepatology. London: BMJ Publications; 1999. p. 305–21.
[45] Craxì A, Di Bona D, Camma C. Interferon-alpha for HBeAg-positive chronic hepatitis B. J Hepatol 2003;39:S99–105 [review].
[46] Papatheodoridis GV, Manesis E, Hadziyannis SJ. The long-term outcome of interferon-alpha treated and untreated patients with HBeAg-negative chronic hepatitis B. J Hepatol 2001;34: 306–13.
[47] Lin SM, Sheen IS, Chien RN, et al. Long-term beneficial effect of interferon therapy in patients with chronic hepatitis B virus infection. Hepatology 1999;29:971–5.
[48] Yuen MF, Hui CK, Cheng CC, et al. Long-term follow-up of interferon alfa treatment in Chinese patients with chronic hepatitis B infection: The effect on hepatitis B e antigen seroconversion and the development of cirrhosis-related complications. Hepatology 2001;34: 139–45.
[49] Niederau C, Heintges T, Lange S, et al. Long-term follow-up of HBeAg-positive patients treated with interferon alfa for chronic hepatitis B. N Engl J Med 1996;334:1422–7.
[50] Di Marco V, Lo Iacono O, Camma C, et al. The long-term course of chronic hepatitis B. Hepatology 1999;30:257–64.
[51] Chen DK, Yim C, O'Rourke K, et al. Long-term follow-up of a randomized trial of interferon therapy for chronic hepatitis B in a predominantly homosexual male population. J Hepatol 1999;30:557–63.
[52] Evans AA, Fine M, London WT. Spontaneous seroconversion in hepatitis B e antigen-positive chronic hepatitis B: implications for interferon therapy. J Infect Dis 1997;176:845–50.
[53] Korenman J, Baker B, Waggoner J, et al. Long-term remission of chronic hepatitis B after alpha-interferon therapy. Ann Intern Med 1991;114:629–34.
[54] Lok AS, Chung HT, Liu VW, et al. Long-term follow-up of chronic hepatitis B patients treated with interferon alfa. Gastroenterology 1993;105:1833–8.
[55] Lau DT, Everhart J, Kleiner DE, et al. Long-term follow-up of patients with chronic hepatitis B treated with interferon alfa. Gastroenterology 1997;113:1660–7.
[56] Fattovich G, Giustina G, Christensen E, et al. Influence of hepatitis delta virus infection on morbidity and mortality in compensated cirrhosis type B. The European Concerted Action on Viral Hepatitis (Eurohep). Gut 2000;46:420–6.
[57] Hsu YS, Chien RN, Yeh CT, et al. Long-term outcome after spontaneous HBeAg seroconversion in patients with chronic hepatitis B. Hepatology 2002;35:1522–7.

[58] Esteban R. Management of chronic hepatitis B: an overview. Semin Liver Dis 2002;22:1–6.
[59] Liaw YF, Sung JJY, Chow WC, et al. Effects of lamivudine on disease progression and development of liver cancer in advanced chronic hepatitis B: a prospective double-blind placebo-controlled clinical trial. Hepatology 2003;38:262A.
[60] Di Marco V, Marzano P, Lampertico P, et al. Virological and clinical events during lamivudine therapy for anti-HBE/HBV-DNA positive chronic liver disease. Hepatology 2004;40:883–91.
[61] Cammà C, Di Marco V, Orlando A, et al. Treatment of small hepatocellular carcinoma with radio-frequency thermal ablation (rfta): a prognostic model. Dig Liver Dis 2004;36:26A.
[62] Orlando A, D'Antoni A, Camma C, et al. Treatment of small hepatocellular carcinoma with percutaneous ethanol injection: a validated prognostic model. Am J Gastroenterol 2000; 95:2921–7.
[63] Lencioni RA, Allgaier HP, Cioni D, et al. Small hepatocellular carcinoma in cirrhosis: randomized comparison of radio-frequency thermal ablation versus percutaneous ethanol injection. Radiology 2003;228:235–40.
[64] Cammà C, Schepis F, Orlando A, et al. Transarterial chemoembolization for unresectable hepatocellular carcinoma: meta-analysis of randomized controlled trials. Radiology 2002;224: 47–54.
[65] Muto Y, Moriwaki H, Ninomiya M, et al. Prevention of second primary tumors by an acyclic retinoid, polyprenoic acid,in patients with hepatocellular carcinoma. Hepatoma Prevention Study Group. N Engl J Med 1996;334:1561–7.
[66] Lau WY, Leung TW, Ho SK, et al. Adjuvant intra-arterial iodine-131-labelled lipiodol for resectablehepatocellular carcinoma: a prospective randomised trial. Lancet 1999;353:797–801.
[67] Takayama T, Sekine T, Makuuchi M, et al. Adoptive immunotherapy to lower postsurgical recurrence rates of hepatocellularcarcinoma: a randomised trial. Lancet 2000;356:802–7.
[68] Ikeda K, Arase Y, Saitoh S, et al. Interferon beta prevents recurrence of hepatocellular carcinoma after completeresection or ablation of the primary tumor—a prospective randomized study of hepatitis C virus-related liver cancer. Hepatology 2000;32:228–32.
[69] Kubo S, Nishiguchi S, Hirohashi K, et al. Randomized clinical trial of long-term outcome after resection of hepatitis C virus-related hepatocellular carcinoma by postoperative interferon therapy. Br J Surg 2002;89:418–22.
[70] Suou T, Mitsuda A, Koda M, et al. Interferon alpha inhibits intrahepatic recurrence in hepatocellular carcinoma with chronic hepatitis C: a pilot study. Hepatol Res 2001;20:301–11.
[71] Miyaguchi S, Watanabe T, Takahashi H, et al. Interferon therapy for hepatocellular carcinoma patients with low HCV-RNA levels. Hepatogastroenterology 2002;49:724–9.
[72] Shiratori Y, Shiina S, Teratani T, et al. Interferon therapy after tumor ablation improves prognosis in patients with hepatocellular carcinoma associated with hepatitis C virus. Ann Intern Med 2003;138:299–306.
[73] Okuno M, Kojima S, Matsushima-Nishiwaki R, et al. Retinoids in cancer chemoprevention. Curr Cancer Drug Targets 2004;4:285–98.
[74] Kojima S, Okuno M, Matsushima-Nishiwaki R, et al. Acyclic retinoid in the chemoprevention of hepatocellular carcinoma. Int J Oncol 2004;24:797–805.

ELSEVIER
SAUNDERS

CLINICS IN
LIVER DISEASE

Clin Liver Dis 9 (2005) 347–351

# Index

*Note:* Page numbers of article titles are in **boldface** type.



1089-3261/05/$ – see front matter 
doi:10.1016/S1089-3261(05)00027-9

## H

# *Changing Your Address?*

Make sure your subscription changes too! When you notify us of your new address, you can help make our job easier by including an exact copy of your Clinics label number with your old address (see illustration below.) This number identifies you to our computer system and will speed the processing of your address change. Please be sure this label number accompanies your old address and your corrected address—you can send an old Clinics label with your number on it or just copy it exactly and send it to the address listed below.

We appreciate your help in our attempt to give you continuous coverage. Thank you.

**W. B. Saunders Company**
SHIPPING AND RECEIVING DEPTS.
151 BENIGNO BLVD.
BELLMAWR, N.J. 08031

SECOND CLASS POSTAGE
**PAID AT BELLMAWR, N.J.**

**This is your copy of the**
**__________ CLINICS OF NORTH AMERICA**

00503570 DOE—J32400    101    NH    8102

JOHN C DOE MD
324 SAMSON ST
BERLIN    NH    03570

XP-D11494

JAN ISSUE

## Your Clinics Label Number

Copy it exactly or send your label along with your address to:
**W.B. Saunders Company, Customer Service**
Orlando, FL 32887-4800
Call Toll Free 1-800-654-2452

Please allow four to six weeks for delivery of new subscriptions and for processing address changes.